Acute Stroke Treatment

Editor: Amitabh Prakash

Adis International
Auckland • Buenos Aires • Chester • Hong Kong • Madrid • Milan • Osaka • Paris • Philadelphia • São Paulo • Sydney

Acute Stroke Treatment

Editor: Amitabh Prakash

A Wolters Kluwer Company

Publication Manager: Lorna Venter-Lewis
Commercial Manager: Gordon Mallarkey
Adis International Limited

Earlier versions of some articles in this book were published in Adis International's peer-reviewed medical journals. The editor has collated the articles and worked with the authors to adapt and update the information for this publication.

Printed in Hong Kong.

Foreword

Acute ischaemic stroke is a leading cause of death and a major cause of disability worldwide.

It is important to limit the extent of stroke damage. This can be achieved by using the most appropriate drugs within a short period of time after stroke has occurred.

This book reviews current treatments for stroke. It looks at the role of stroke units and the place of clinical guidelines in maximising the outcome of stroke management. Combined with this strong clinical focus, there is also an in-depth look at the cost of stroke.

Dr Amitabh Prakash
Editor
Drugs & Aging

March 2000

Dr Prakash is Editor of ***Drugs & Aging****, an international journal that reviews clinical pharmacology and disease management in elderly patients. Age-related physiological changes with clinical implications for drug therapy also fall within the scope of the journal.*

Acute Stroke Treatment

Contents

Limiting Neurological Damage after Stroke

A Review of Pharmacological Treatment Options

Stephen J. Read,[1,3] *Teruyuki Hirano,*[1] *Stephen M. Davis*[2,3] and *Geoffrey A. Donnan*[1,3]

1 Department of Neurology, Austin and Repatriation Medical Centre, Heidelberg, Victoria, Australia

2 Department of Neurology, Royal Melbourne Hospital, Melbourne, Victoria, Australia

3 Department of Medicine, University of Melbourne, Melbourne, Victoria, Australia

1. Cellular Events Leading to Brain Tissue Injury Following Ischaemic Stroke: Rationale for Pharmacological Intervention

Astrup and colleagues were the first to develop the concept of the ischaemic penumbra and to suggest that acute ischaemic stroke was a potentially treatable disease.[1] Using a baboon model of focal ischaemia they demonstrated that tissues exhibited failure of electrical function at a higher level of cerebral blood flow (CBF) [approximately 16 ml/100g/min] than that at which they exhibited membrane failure, with failure of membrane Na^+-K^+-ATPase resulting in release of K^+ from cells and membrane depolarisation (approximately 10 ml/ 100g/min). They also showed that tissue with CBF between these thresholds was potentially salvageable, as electrical function could be restored if ischaemia was reversed.[2] They termed tissues with CBF between the thresholds of electrical and membrane failure the 'ischaemic penumbra'.

The existence of penumbral tissues after ischaemic stroke is a result of the nature of focal ischaemia. The degree of hypoperfusion in the ischaemic territory varies from the centre, which receives little collateral blood supply and is most severely ischaemic (the infarct core), to the peripheries, which are less severely ischaemic because of better collateral blood supply. As the duration of tissue survival is inversely proportional to the severity of ischaemia,[3] it is these peripheral areas which survive longest and largely comprise the ischaemic penumbra.

How long penumbral tissues survive, and thus the duration of the therapeutic window after stroke, has not been established in humans. Using positron emission tomography (PET) to measure CBF, the rate of cerebral oxygen metabolism ($CMRO_2$) and raised oxygen extraction fraction (OEF), and defining the penumbra as tissue with reduced CBF, relatively preserved $CMRO_2$ and raised OEF, penumbral tissues have been detected in the peripheries of ischaemia up to 72 hours post-stroke.[4,5] They may comprise a significant proportion of the final volume of infarction (up to 50%) as late as 17 hours post-stroke,[6] but most of the penumbra generally undergoes progressive metabolic derangement and infarction during the 2 to 3 weeks after stroke.[5] The outcome for patients after stroke is related to the proportion of penumbral tissue which survives the ischaemic insult.[7] Hence, therapies that preserve or salvage penumbral tissues should improve clinical outcomes for patients who have experienced a stroke.

The eventual demise of much of the penumbra is due to a complex cascade of events which follows the onset of ischaemia (fig. 1). Ischaemia impairs cellular energy production, and

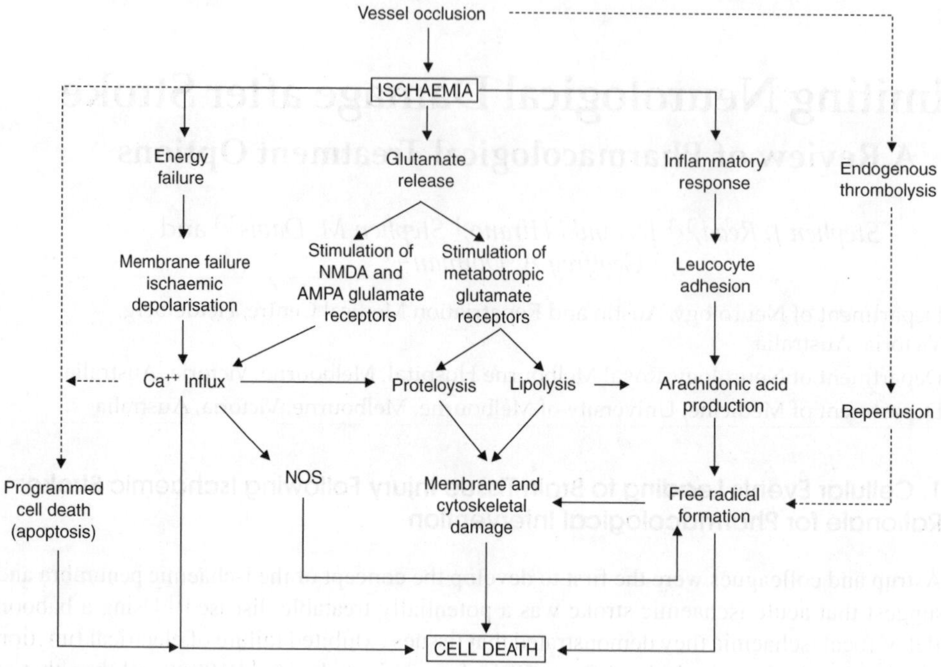

Fig. 1. A simplified diagram of the sequence of events that may lead to cell death after the onset of cerebral ischaemia. **AMPA** = α-amino-3-hydroxy-5-methyl-4-isoxazole propionic acid; **NMDA** = *N*-methyl-D-aspartate; **NOS** = nitric oxide synthase.

depletion of adenosine triphosphate (ATP) in turn impairs cellular membrane function and ionic homeostasis by interfering with the Na^+-K^+-ATPase. Initially, at milder levels of ischaemia, this manifests as cell swelling (cytotoxic oedema), which forms the basis for the detection of acute stroke using diffusion-weighted magnetic resonance imaging (DWI).[8] At more severe levels, around 10 ml/100g/min CBF, failure of Na^+-K^+-ATPase function occurs, with K^+ efflux from and calcium ion (Ca^{++}) influx into cells.[9,10] This ischaemic depolarisation is accompanied by uncontrolled release of neurotransmitters, most notably the excitatory amino acid glutamate.[11-13] When glutamate is released from presynaptic endings, it activates two postsynaptic receptor types that are linked to ion channels: the *N*-methyl-D-aspartate (NMDA) receptor [which allows sodium ion (Na^+) and Ca^{++} influx and K^+ efflux] and the α-amino-3-hydroxy-5-methyl-4-isoxazole propionic acid (AMPA) receptor [which allows Na^+ influx and K^+ efflux] (fig. 2). Massive release of glutamate thus causes depolarisation of adjacent neurons, triggering further neurotransmitter release, increasing their energy requirements and tipping them into energy failure. This is the basis of so-called 'excitotoxic cell injury'.[14]

Depolarisation, whether induced by energy failure or by glutamate, is accompanied by Ca^{++} influx. Ca^{++} enters the cell either via agonist- or receptor-operated calcium channels, mainly gated by NMDA receptors, or via voltage-gated calcium channels (VGCCs), activated when Na^+ influx leads to depolarisation. VGCCs of the L- and T-types occur on postsynaptic membranes, while those of the N-, P- and Q-types occur on presynaptic membranes. The L- and T-types are involved in regulating neurotransmitter release in response to depolarisation.[15]

Movement of Ca^{++} from the extracellular to the intracellular space and release of these ions from internal stores triggers activation of enzymes [proteases, phospholipases, endonucleases, protein kinases, nitric oxide synthase (NOS), etc.], which may affect the structure and function of a variety of cellular constituents (membrane ion channels, receptors, cytoskeletal elements, etc.)[16] [fig. 2].

Glutamate also stimulates metabotropic receptors, resulting in activation of phospholipases [especially phospholipase C (PLC) and phospholipase A_2 (PLA_2)].[17,18] PLC cleaves phosphatidylinositol biphosphate (PIP_2), yielding inositol triphosphate (IP_3) and diacylglycerol (DAG).[16,17] IP_3 triggers the release of Ca^{++} from internal stores (so-called 'calciosomes', including the endoplasmic reticulum) [fig. 2].[17] Hydrolysis of membrane

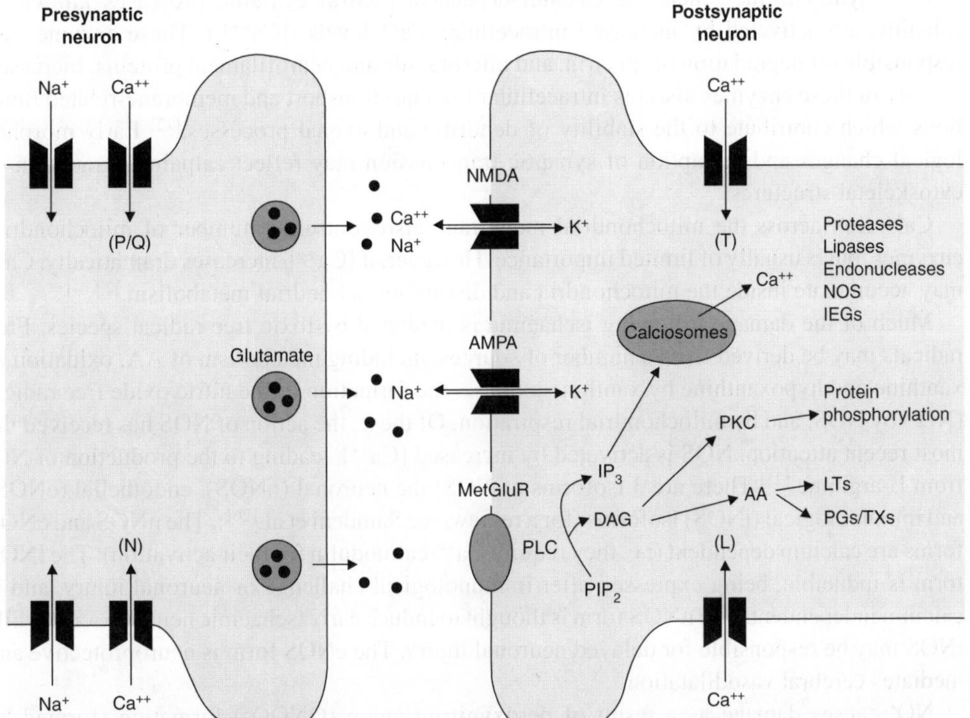

Fig. 2. Schematic diagram illustrating pre- and postsynaptic ion channels. Presynaptically, the voltage-sensitive calcium channels (VSCC) involved in transmitter release are assumed to be of the N-, P- and Q-type, whereas the L- and T-types are assumed to be localised to dendrites and cell bodies. Release of the excitatory transmitter glutamate is shown to activate 2 types of receptors, the *N*-methyl-D-aspartate (NMDA) and the α-amino-3-hydroxy-5-methyl-4-isoxazole propionic acid (AMPA) receptors. The AMPA receptor gates a channel that is permeable to Na^+, K^+ and H^+, while the NMDA receptor is also permeable to Ca^{++} ions. Glutamate also stimulates metabotropic receptors (MetGluR), resulting in activation of phospholipase C (PLC). PLC cleaves phosphatidylinositol biphosphate (PIP_2), yielding inositol triphosphate (IP_3) and diacylglycerol (DAG). IP_3 triggers Ca^{++} release from internal stores, calciosomes. Activation of PLC provides substrate for the production of arachidonic acid (AA). AA gives rise to eicosanoids [prostaglandins (PGs) and thromboxanes (TXs) via the cyclooxygenase pathway, and leukotrienes (LTs) via the lipoxygenase pathway]. Accumulation of DAG also activates protein kinase C (PKC), leading to protein phosphorylation which affects ion channel and receptor activity.
IEGs = immediate-early genes; **NOS** = nitric oxide synthase .

phospholipids damages the cell membrane and results in the release of free fatty acids and lysophospholipids which are themselves toxic. Activation of PLC and PLA_2 provides substrate for the production of arachidonic acid (AA).[16] AA potentiates NMDA receptor currents,[19] blocks γ-aminobutyric acid (GABA)–induced neuronal inhibition,[20] and gives rise to the eicosanoids (prostaglandins and thromboxanes via the cyclooxygenase pathway, and leukotrienes via the lipoxygenase pathway) [fig. 2]. Activation of PLA_2 also results in increased levels of platelet activating factor (PAF), which can alter membrane function and act as a chemoattractant.[16] Accumulation of DAG also activates protein kinase C (PKC), leading to protein phosphorylation and affecting ion channel and receptor activity, although this activation is transient.[21] DNA-related events, such as immediate–early gene expression and protein synthesis, are also triggered.[16]

Proteolytic enzymes, including calcium–dependent neutral cysteine proteases known as calpains, are activated by increased intracellular Ca^{++} levels ($[Ca^{++}]_i$). These enzymes are responsible for degradation of spectrin, and microtubule and neurofilament proteins. Increased activity of these enzymes disrupts intracellular (axonal) transport and membrane-related functions which contribute to the stability of dendritic and axonal processes.[22] Early morphological changes and disruption of synaptic transmission may reflect calpain degradation of cytoskeletal structures.

Ca^{++} flux across the mitochondrial membrane also controls a number of mitochondrial enzymes, but is usually of limited importance. However, if $[Ca^{++}]_i$ increases dramatically, Ca^{++} may accumulate inside the mitochondria and disrupt mitochondrial metabolism.[23,24]

Much of the damage following ischaemia is mediated by toxic free radical species. Free radicals may be derived from a number of sources, including metabolism of AA, oxidation of xanthine and hypoxanthine by xanthine oxidase, the formation of the nitric oxide free radical ($NO^{\bullet}$) by NOS, and by mitochondrial respiration. Of these, the action of NOS has received the most recent attention. NOS is activated by increased $[Ca^{++}]_i$ leading to the production of $NO^{\bullet}$ from L-arginine.[25] There are 3 isoforms of NOS: the neuronal (nNOS), endothelial (eNOS) and immunological (iNOS) isoforms (for a review, see Samdeni et al.[26]). The nNOS and eNOS forms are calcium dependent (i.e. they require Ca^{++}/calmodulin for their activation). The iNOS form is inducible, being expressed after immunological challenge or neuronal injury, and is calcium independent. The nNOS form is thought to induce early ischaemic neurotoxicity, while iNOS may be responsible for delayed neuronal injury. The eNOS form is neuroprotective and mediates cerebral vasodilatation.

$NO^{\bullet}$ causes damage as a result of peroxynitrite anion ($ONOO^-$) formation (formed by combination with the superoxide free radical anion [$O_2^{\bullet -}$]). $ONOO^-$ causes lipid peroxidation and depletion of energy stores by activation of poly(ADP-ribose) synthase.[27,28] Usually $O_2^{\bullet -}$ is rapidly scavenged by superoxide dismutase (SOD), but if $NO^{\bullet}$ production is rapid, as in reperfusion, it competes with SOD for $O_2^{\bullet -}$ and $ONOO^-$ is formed.

Reperfusion, whether by endogenous thrombolysis, embolus migration or therapeutic intervention, may aggravate ischaemic damage. Free radical formation is increased in reperfused tissues, and cytokine release during ischaemia leads to leucocyte adhesion and activation in the reperfused tissues. Leucocyte adhesion may cause mechanical occlusion of the microvasculature (contributing to the 'no-reflow' phenomenon), further free radical generation, release of proteases causing endothelial injury and tissue invasion leading ultimately to necrosis.[29]

Table I. Drugs undergoing clinical evaluation for the treatment of stroke

Mechanism	Drug	Efficacy	Current status
Thrombolysis	Alteplase	Effective	Approved in USA; under regulatory review elsewhere
	Streptokinase	Ineffective at doses tested	Further trials at lower doses may be warranted
Antithrombotics	Heparin	Ineffective	
	LMWH	Ineffective	
	Heparinoids	Ineffective	
Antiplatelet agents	Aspirin (acetylsalicylic acid)	Equivocal results; prevents early recurrence only	
Calcium antagonists	Nimodipine	Ineffective; results pending for use <12h after the onset of symptoms	Trials ongoing in which the drug is admininstered <12h after the onset of symptoms (VENUS)
NMDA antagonists	Selfotel	Ineffective	Development discontinued (due to safety concerns)
	Aptiganel	Equivocal results	Development discontinued (due to safety concerns)
	Dextrorphan	Results pending	Development discontinued
	Dextromethorphan	Results pending	Trials ongoing
	Remacemide	Results pending	Phase II trials ongoing
	Magnesium	Results pending	Phase III trial (IMAGES) ongoing
	Eliprodil	Results pending	Development discontinued
	GV-150526A	Results pending	Phase II trials ongoing
	ACEA 1021	Results pending	Phase II trials ongoing
Glutamate release inhibitors	Fosphenytoin	Results pending	Phase II trials ongoing
	Lubeluzole	Equivocal results	Development discontinued
	Lifarizine	Equivocal results	Development discontinued
Free radical scavengers	Tirilazad	Ineffective	Development discontinued
Opioid antagonists	Nalmefene	Results pending	Phase II trials ongoing
Gangliosides	GM-1	Ineffective	Development discontinued
Growth factors	bFGF	Results pending	Nth American trial ceased (due to safety concerns); European/Australian trial ongoing
Antiadhesion molecules	ICAM	Ineffective	
GABA agonists	Clomethiazole	Ineffective	
Nootropic agents	Piracetam	Eqivocal results	Further phase III studies ongoing with administration of the drug <7h after the onset of symptoms

bFGF = basic fibroblast growth factor; **ECASS** = European Cooperative Acute Stroke Study; **GABA** = γ-aminobutyric acid; **ICAM** = intercellular adhesion molecule; **IMAGES** = Intravenous Magnesium Efficacy in Stroke Trial; **LMWH** = low molecular weight heparins; **NMDA** = *N*-methyl-D aspartate; **VENUS** = Very Early Nimodipine Use in Stroke study.

Cell death following ischaemia thus results from the accumulated damaging effects of this complicated cascade of metabolic/biochemical events that impair cell function. One additional mode of cell death is the activation of apoptosis, or 'programmed cell death'. Apoptosis is a process by which a cell, in response to a stimulus, activates a controlled cascade of intracellular events that leads to its own death. Whilst the exact trigger for apoptosis remains to be determined, it appears to follow Ca^{++} influx,[30] and to contribute to the increase in infarct volume observed over the days to weeks following stroke.

It can be seen that, within this complex cascade of events, there are a number of points where pharmacological agents can potentially be used to reduce the damaging effects of ischaemia. In sections 2 and 3, we review the drugs which have been assessed in animal models of ischaemia and in clinical trials. A list of drug classes and representative examples of agents currently undergoing clinical evaluation are given in table I.

2. Thrombolytic and Antithrombotic Therapy

2.1 Thrombolytics

Thrombolytic agents are an attractive option as therapy for acute stroke because timely reperfusion of the ischaemic territory is likely to achieve maximum tissue salvage. While thrombolytic agents were first tested as stroke therapy in the late 1950s, early results were disappointing and trials were hampered by the inability to reliably distinguish ischaemic from haemorrhagic stroke (thrombolytics being contraindicated in the latter. Evidence from various experimental stroke models that thrombolytic agents could minimise the effects of ischaemia,[31] together with the advent of modern neuroimaging techniques, has provided the impetus for the re-evaluation of thrombolytic therapy in acute ischaemic stroke.

2.1.1 Intravenous Administration

Streptokinase and Alteplase

After some small trials showed promising results,[32-36] five major trials of thrombolytics were mounted during the early 1990s.[37-41] Three of these involved the administration of streptokinase[37-39] and two involved the use of alteplase (tissue plasminogen activator).[40,41] All three streptokinase trials were stopped prematurely because of concerns raised by the Safety Monitoring Committee of one of the studies, the Multicentre Acute Stroke Trial – Europe (MAST-E).[37] In this study, early mortality was increased because of an excess of fatal haemorrhagic stroke in the treatment group. In the Australian Streptokinase Trial (ASK) a similar pattern emerged in the subset of patients who received therapy more than 3 hours after the onset of symptoms, but this pattern was not seen in those patients receiving therapy in the 0- to 3-hour time window.[38] However, because of the impracticality of continuing the study, recruitment was stopped and the results published.

The trials of alteplase were somewhat more promising. The European Cooperative Acute Stroke Study (ECASS)[40] assessed 620 patients aged 18 to 80 years who had presented with a stable, moderate-to-severe, hemispheric stroke syndrome, and who had no or only minor early infarct signs as determined by computerised tomography (CT). Patients were randomised within 6 hours of onset to either alteplase given as a single intravenous dose of 1.1 mg/kg or placebo. On an intention-to-treat analysis, there was no difference between the treatment and placebo groups with respect to the primary outcome measures of Barthel Index and modified Rankin Scale at 90 days or in secondary end-points, including 30-day mortality. A 'target population' analysis was also performed, in which 109 patients who had been randomised despite early CT changes (i.e. in violation of the study protocol) were excluded. A significant improvement in measures of neurological recovery at 90 days was seen with alteplase treatment in this analysis. Alteplase therapy was associated with a significant excess of parenchymal haemorrhage (19.8% with active drug *vs* 6.5% with placebo). This excess of haemorrhage was greatest in the patients treated with the drug despite early CT signs of infarction and was associated with a nonsignificant excess mortality.

In the National Institute of Neurological Disorders and Stroke (NINDS) trial,[41] a somewhat more aggressive approach to early recruitment was taken. A time window for initiating therapy of no more than 3 hours after the onset of symptoms was chosen, and almost half of the 632 patients randomised were recruited within 90 minutes of symptom onset. A single intravenous dose of alteplase 0.9 mg/kg was used and all subtypes of ischaemic stroke were considered for entry with no restrictions based on severity or CT appearances (other than the absence of haemorrhage). Compared with patients receiving placebo, those treated with alteplase were 30% more likely to have no disability or only minor neurological impairment at 3 months post-stroke, but there was no difference in mortality between the two groups. Importantly, there was an approximately 6% symptomatic cerebral haemorrhage rate among those who received alteplase. Based on the results of this trial, alteplase was approved in the US as therapy for acute ischaemic stroke if given within 3 hours of stroke onset and under the guidelines established by the NINDS trial investigators.

Following publication of these studies, a meta-analysis of all trials of intravenous thrombolytic therapy was performed.[42] It showed an overall benefit for thrombolytic therapy (fig. 3), especially for therapy with altepase. However, this benefit comes at the risk of increased mortality, predominantly caused by increased rates of cerebral haemorrhage (fig. 4).

Persisting uncertainty regarding the effectiveness of altepase, the optimal dose and the time window during which therapy might be effective led to the ECASS II trial.[49] 800 patients with ischaemic stroke were randomised to a single intravenous dose of 0.9 mg/kg of altepase

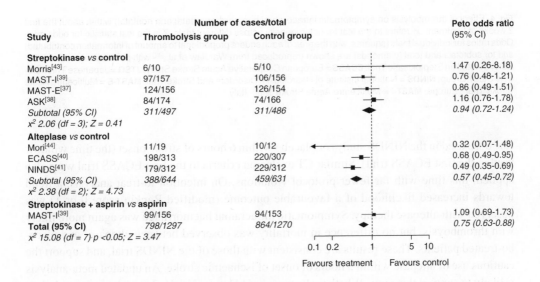

Study	Number of cases/total: Thrombolysis group	Control group	Peto odds ratio (95% CI)
Streptokinase *vs* control			
Morris[43]	6/10	5/10	1.47 (0.26-8.18)
MAST-I[39]	97/157	106/156	0.76 (0.48-1.21)
MAST-E[37]	124/156	126/154	0.86 (0.49-1.51)
ASK[38]	84/174	74/166	1.16 (0.76-1.78)
Subtotal (95% CI)	*311/497*	*311/486*	*0.94 (0.72-1.24)*
x^2 2.06 (df = 3); Z = 0.41			
Alteplase *vs* control			
Mori[44]	11/19	10/12	0.32 (0.07-1.48)
ECASS[40]	198/313	220/307	0.68 (0.49-0.95)
NINDS[41]	179/312	229/312	0.49 (0.35-0.69)
Subtotal (95% CI)	*388/644*	*459/631*	*0.57 (0.45-0.72)*
x^2 2.38 (df = 2); Z = 4.73			
Streptokinase + aspirin *vs* aspirin			
MAST-I[39]	99/156	94/153	1.09 (0.69-1.73)
Total (95% CI)	*798/1297*	*864/1270*	*0.75 (0.63-0.88)*
x^2 15.08 (df = 7) p <0.05; Z = 3.47			

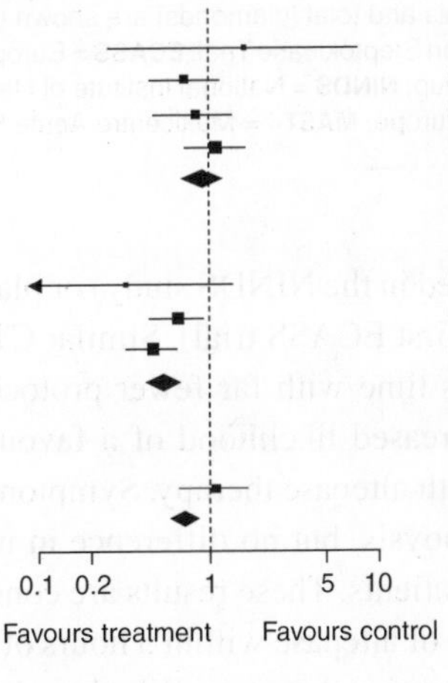

Fig. 3. Effect of thrombolysis on death or dependency at the end of trial follow-up. x^2 refers to the test for heterogeneity across different trials. Z is the test statistic for odds ratio. Odds ratios for individual trials (squares, with the area of each square proportional to the amount of information contributed) and for subtotals and total (diamonds) are shown (reproduced from Wardlaw et al.,[42] with permission).
ASK = Australian Steptokinase Trial; **ECASS** = European Cooperative Acute Stroke Study; **NINDS** = National Institute of Neurological Disorders and Stroke Trial ; **MAST-E** = Multicentre Acute Stroke Trial - Europe; **MAST-I** = Multicentre Acute Stroke Trial - Italy.

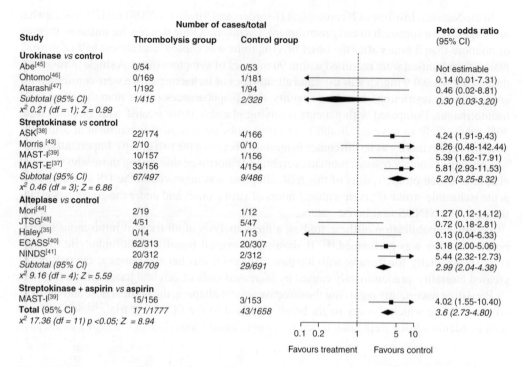

Study	Number of cases/total: Thrombolysis group	Control group	Peto odds ratio (95% CI)
Urokinase *vs* control			
Abe[45]	0/54	0/53	Not estimable
Ohtomo[46]	0/169	1/181	0.14 (0.01-7.31)
Atarashi[47]	1/192	1/94	0.46 (0.02-8.81)
Subtotal (95% CI)	*1/415*	*2/328*	*0.30 (0.03-3.20)*
x^2 0.21 (df = 1); Z = 0.99			
Streptokinase *vs* control			
ASK[38]	22/174	4/166	4.24 (1.91-9.43)
Morris [43]	2/10	0/10	8.26 (0.48-142.44)
MAST-I[39]	10/157	1/156	5.39 (1.62-17.91)
MAST-E[37]	33/156	4/154	5.81 (2.93-11.53)
Subtotal (95% CI)	*67/497*	*9/486*	*5.20 (3.25-8.32)*
x^2 0.46 (df = 3); Z = 6.86			
Alteplase *vs* control			
Mori[44]	2/19	1/12	1.27 (0.12-14.12)
JTSG[48]	4/51	5/47	0.72 (0.18-2.81)
Haley[35]	0/14	1/13	0.13 (0.04-6.33)
ECASS[40]	62/313	20/307	3.18 (2.00-5.06)
NINDS[41]	20/312	2/312	5.44 (2.32-12.73)
Subtotal (95% CI)	*88/709*	*29/691*	*2.99 (2.04-4.38)*
x^2 9.16 (df = 4); Z = 5.59			
Streptokinase + aspirin *vs* aspirin			
MAST-I[39]	15/156	3/153	4.02 (1.55-10.40)
Total (95% CI)	*171/1777*	*43/1658*	*3.6 (2.73-4.80)*
x^2 17.36 (df = 11) p <0.05; Z = 8.94			

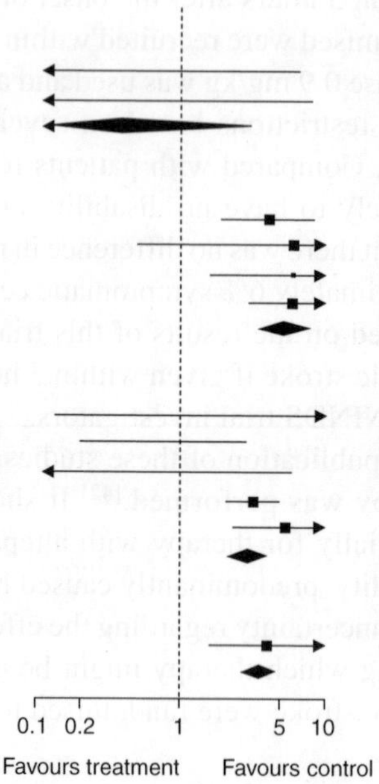

Fig. 4. Effect of thrombolysis on symptomatic intracerebral haemorrhage (fatal and nonfatal) within about the first 2 weeks of treatment. x^2 refers to the test for heterogeneity across different trials. Z is the test statistic for odds ratio. Odds ratios for individual trials (squares, with the area of each square proportional to amount of information contributed) and for subtotals and total (diamonds) are shown (reproduced from Wardlaw et al.,[42] with permission).
ASK = Australian Steptokinase Trial; **ECASS** = European Cooperative Acute Stroke Study; **JTSG** = Japanese Thrombolysis Study Group; **NINDS** = National Institute of Neurological Disorders and Stroke Trial; **MAST-E** = Multicentre Acute Stroke Trial - Europe; **MAST-I** = Multicentre Acute Stroke Trial - Italy.

(the dose used in the NINDS study) or placebo within 6 hours of stroke onset (the time window used in the first ECASS trial). Similar CT exclusion criteria to the first ECASS trial were also applied, this time with far fewer protocol violations. On intention-to-treat analysis, a trend towards increased likelihood of a favourable outcome (modified Rankin score 0 or 1) was observed with altepase therapy. Symptomatic intracranial haemorrhage was again more likely with thromboysis, but no difference in mortality was observed between altepase- and placebo-treated patients. These results are consistent with those of the NINDS trial, and support the cautious use of altepase within 3 hours of onset of ischaemic stroke. An updated meta-analysis is likely to support this view. Whether altepase should be used in the 3- to 6-hour time window is still unclear.

2.1.2 Intra-Arterial Administration

The intra-arterial administration of fibrinolytic agents has been studied since the early 1980s, with the expectation that this route of administration would result in superior recanalisation rates to those achieved with intravenous administration.[50-52] Initially, the fibrinolytic agent was delivered into the cervical carotid or vertebral arteries (regional administration); later, to achieve delivery of higher concentrations to the thrombus, administration via a microcatheter positioned in an intracranial cerebral artery (local administration) was used. None of these early studies were randomised controlled trials, but all suggested that intra-arterial thrombolysis was indeed well tolerated and efficacious.

Results of the first double-blind, randomised, placebo-controlled study of intra-arterial administration of a plasminogen activator [the Prolyse in Acute Cerebral Thromboembolism (PROACT) trial] have recently been published.[53] After clinical and angiographic screening to select patients for therapy, 40 patients were treated with either a single dose of pro-urokinase 6mg (n = 26) or placebo (n = 14) within 6 hours of stroke onset. Recanalisation of documented M1 or M2 occlusion at 120 minutes after treatment was significantly more frequent with pro-urokinase therapy (57.7 *vs* 14.3% with placebo; $2p = 0.017$). There was no significant difference in the frequency of cerebral haemorrhage causing neurological deterioration between the active drug and placebo groups at 24 hours or 90 days. Although this result is promising, intra-arterial thrombolysis is more time consuming than intravenous therapy and not available at every hospital. Further analysis of the risks and the benefits of this approach are required.

2.2 Antithrombotic Therapy

The use of heparins or heparinoids in acute ischaemic stroke is based on the assumption that they may inhibit clot propagation within small and large arteries associated with the ischaemic area and also prevent early arterial re-embolisation. Further, they might be expected to reduce the risk of venous thromboembolism, given evidence from other studies where limbs have been immobilised[54-57]. However, there is little or no experimental evidence to support the use of these agents after acute ischaemic stroke in spite of their routine clinical use for this indication in many countries. A number of large clinical studies have now been performed to test the hypothesis that heparins or heparinoids improve outcomes if administered early after the onset of ischaemic stroke.

The largest of these studies, the International Stroke Trial (IST),[58] was a factorially designed trial in which patients with all forms of ischaemic stroke were randomised to receive either unfractionated heparin (in one of 2 doses; 5000 or 12500IU twice daily subcutaneously) or no heparin, and either aspirin (acetylsalicylic acid) [300mg daily] or no aspirin. Treatment was to begin within 48 hours of stroke onset and to continue for 14 days or until prior discharge. The results were disappointing in that neither heparin regimen offered any clinical advantage at 6 months. Indeed, the higher dose (12500IU twice daily) was associated with an excess of haemorrhagic strokes and death from any cause within 14 days. Importantly, there was no protection from recurrent ischaemic stroke. There was only a marginally significant reduction in pulmonary embolism with heparin, which was more notable with the higher dose heparin ($2p < 0.05$). Interestingly, the incidence of recurrent ischaemic stroke in the presence of atrial fibrillation was relatively low (4.9%), but was significantly reduced by the use of heparin (2.8%, $2p < 0.01$).

Low molecular weight heparin was used in a pilot study in Hong Kong where patients were randomly assigned within 48 hours of the onset of symptoms to receive one of two dosages of nadroparin calcium (4100 anti-factor Xa IU twice daily, or 4100IU once daily) or placebo subcutaneously for 10 days.[59] Among the 312 patients randomised, there was a significant, dose-dependent effect in favour of low molecular weight heparin ($p = 0.005$, chi squared test for trend). Although the sample size was small, the dose-dependent effect was intriguing enough to warrant mounting a larger study in Europe, Australasia and Hong Kong (FISS-BIS). Here, the time window for therapy was reduced to 24 hours, the sample size increased to 750 and nadroparin calcium used in dosages of 100 IU/kg daily or twice daily for 10 days. This study has now been completed and, while yet to be published, it is understood that the results of this study were negative.

Similarly, the Trial of ORG 10172 in Acute Stroke Treatment (TOAST)[60] randomised 1281 patients to receive either danaparoid sodium (ORG 10172) [bolus followed by infusion adjusted to maintain anti-factor X_a activity at 0.6-0.8 U/ml] or placebo for 7 days, commencing within 24 hours of stroke onset. Disappointingly, there was no difference in primary outcome measures between the 2 groups, although a subgroup analysis was performed and revealed that those patients with a large artery-to-artery mechanism of ischaemic stroke had significantly better outcomes.

In summary, there is currently no evidence that either heparin or heparinoids improve outcomes after acute ischaemic stroke, although the hypothesis-generating information from the TOAST trial may warrant further study in the subgroup of patients with artery-to-artery embolic stroke.

2.3 Antiplatelet Agents

As for the heparins and heparinoids, there is little experimental evidence to support the view that antiplatelet agents are likely to minimise the volume of infarction after the onset of vessel occlusion or improve clinical outcomes. However, because of their proven role in secondary prevention and the theoretical benefit which may be accrued from prevention of clot propagation, aspirin has been studied on a number of occasions as a potential form of acute stroke therapy.

The Chinese Acute Stroke Trial (CAST)[61] was a large randomised, placebo-controlled trial of the effects, in hospital, of aspirin treatment (160mg daily) started within 48 hours of the onset of acute ischaemic stroke and continued in hospital for up to 4 weeks. Outcomes were improved with aspirin therapy in that there was a significant 14% proportional reduction in mortality ($2p = 0.04$), with fewer recurrent ischaemic strokes ($2p = 0.01$) and a significant reduction in the combined in-hospital end-point of

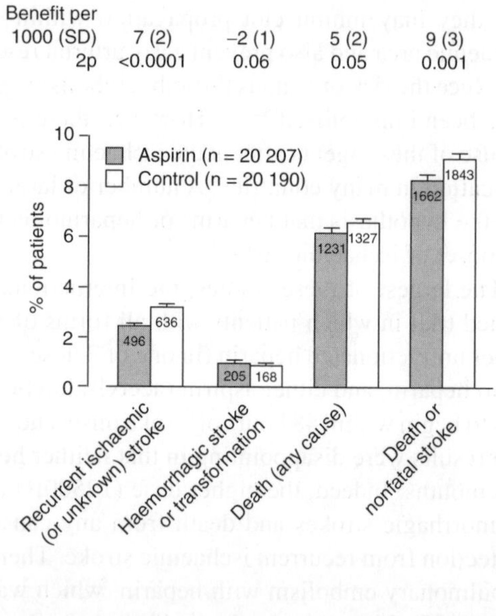

Fig. 5. Overview of the absolute effects of early aspirin (acetylsalicylic acid) treatment in patients with acute ischaemic stroke on clinical events during scheduled treatment periods of the Chinese Acute Stroke Trial (CAST),[61] International Stroke Trial (IST)[58] and Multicentre Acute Stroke Trial - Italy (MAST-I).[39] Numbers in bars indicate actual number of cases. Error bars = 1 standard error for percentage (reproduced from CAST Collaborative Group,[61] with permission). **SD** = standard deviation.

death or nonfatal stroke at 4 weeks (2p = 0.03). However, the absolute difference in the treatment groups of 6.8 deaths or nonfatal strokes per 1000 is not great.

Aspirin was also included in the factorial design of IST (section 2.2). In this study, the effects of immediate aspirin use in acute ischaemic stroke on the unadjusted primary outcomes (death within 14 days and death or dependency at 6 months) were not significant.[58] However, there was a reduction of 11 (± 5) deaths or nonfatal recurrent strokes within 14 days per 1000 patients administered aspirin. It appears, therefore, that much of this early beneficial effect was due to a reduction in early recurrent ischaemic stroke. In other words, an early secondary prevention effect has been shown.

When the data from CAST, IST and MAST-I are aggregated, a modest beneficial effect of aspirin can be seen.[61] There is a significant reduction in recurrent ischaemic stroke, death attributable to any cause, and death or nonfatal stroke. However, this is at the expense of a small increase in haemorrhagic stroke or haemorrhagic transformation (fig. 5). Hence, it can be seen that the biological importance of aspirin usage in acute ischaemic stroke is small but, given the low costs and ease of administration, this may be considered by many to be a useful therapeutic approach for early secondary prevention.

3. Neuroprotective Agents

3.1 Calcium Antagonists

Given the central role of Ca^{++} in mediating ischaemic neuronal damage, drugs that reduce Ca^{++} influx might be expected to be effective stroke therapies.

3.1.1 Nimodipine

Nimodipine, a dihydropyridine compound that blocks L-type calcium channels, is the most extensively studied calcium antagonist in the treatment of cerebral ischaemia. The drug has a selective effect on cerebral vessels and is of established value in the treatment of vasospasm following aneurysmal subarachnoid haemorrhage, whether given intravenously or orally.[62-66] In animal models of cerebral ischaemia, nimodipine reduces the extent of ischaemic damage.[67-70] However, results of clinical trials with oral nimodipine have been conflicting.

In the first large controlled trial, 186 patients were randomised to oral nimodipine (120mg daily for 28 days, begun within 24 hours of stroke onset) or placebo.[71] A reduction in neurological disability and mortality was observed in the treatment group, although the benefits were confined to men. Several trials using similar dosage regimens (120mg daily, begun within 48 hours of stroke onset and continued for 14 to 28 days) subsequently reported negative results.[72-78] The failure to demonstrate efficacy in these trials may be explained by either the delay in initiating treatment (up to 48 hours after symptom onset) in many patients or the deleterious effect of nimodipine-induced hypotension on cerebral perfusion. The former explanation is suggested by the American Nimodipine Study Group[75] in which subgroup analysis revealed that patients treated with nimodipine within 18 hours of stroke onset had a better outcome. The latter explanation is suggested by Kaste et al.[78] who found that a higher early case-fatality rate with nimodipine treatment was associated with a blood pressure–lowering effect.

A meta-analysis of 9 published trials, involving 3719 patients randomised to oral nimodipine or placebo, revealed no significant difference in overall outcome. However, a 38% reduction in the odds of an unfavourable outcome for those treated with nimodipine within 12 hours of symptom onset was found.[79] Conversely, treatment initiated after 24 hours increased the odds of an unfavourable outcome. As a result, early treatment with nimodipine (initiated within 12 hours of stroke onset) is now being evaluated [in the Very Early Nimodipine Use in Stroke (VENUS) study].[80]

While intravenous therapy may be more useful in patients with acute stroke symptoms, trials of intravenous nimodipine have also been disappointing. No benefit[81] or a worse functional outcome[82,83] compared with placebo was reported with a dosage of nimodipine 2 mg/h. Again, this deleterious effect on outcome is thought to be related to nimodipine-induced hypotension. A lower dosage (1 mg/h) resulted in less hypotension, but a trend towards a worse functional outcome was also observed.[83] Bridgers et al.[82] found that functional outcome in patients with moderate deficits as a consequence of their stroke who were treated within 12 hours of stroke onset was significantly improved in those patients who received nimodipine 1 mg/h compared with those who received either placebo or a dosage of 2 mg/h. There is still a need to test a dose of intravenous nimodipine therapy that does not cause hypotension and to assess the most appropriate time window for administration.

3.1.2 Other Calcium Antagonists

Other dihydropyridine calcium antagonists, including isradipine, flunarizine and darodipine (PY-108068), have been assessed in humans but have also proved disappointing, with none producing any significant benefit.[84-88] Compounds acting at other types of calcium channels [in particular N-, P- and Q-types, which are involved in neurotransmitter release from the presynaptic terminal (see section 1)] have been shown to be effective in animal models.[89-91] Human trials with SNX-111 (ziconotide), a synthetic peptide corresponding to ω-conotoxin MVIIA and which inhibits N-type calcium channels, are in progress.

3.2 Glutamate Receptor Antagonists

The adverse effects of the excitatory amino acid neurotransmitter glutamate in stroke might be reduced by blocking one of the glutamate receptor subtypes (NMDA, AMPA, metabotropic or kainate receptors).

3.2.1 N-Methyl-D-Aspartate Receptor Antagonists

NMDA receptors are linked to ion channels for Ca^{++} and Na^{+} and possess binding sites for glutamate, glycine, phencyclidine (PCP), polyamines and magnesium (see fig. 6), all of which can be blocked by specific compounds.

Open Channel Blockers

A number of noncompetitive NMDA receptor antagonists bind to the PCP recognition site in the open NMDA-gated ion channel. Magnesium possesses its own binding site in the ion channel.

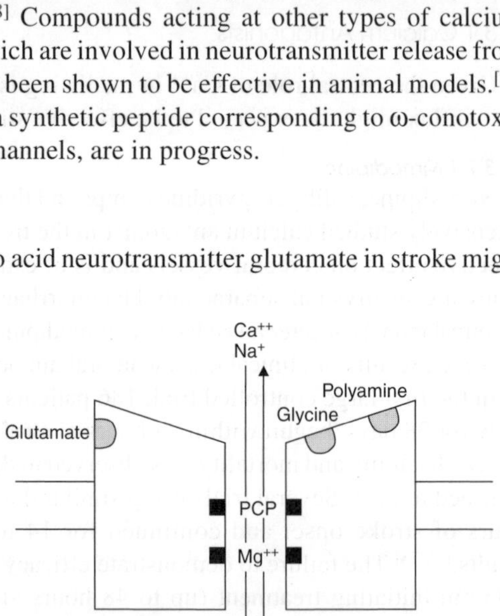

Fig. 6. The *N*-methyl-D-asparate (NMDA) receptor-channel complex. The diagram illustrates the modulators of the receptor complex. Apart from the main recognition site for glutamate, the NMDA receptor contains modulatory sites at which glycine or polyamines act to potentiate the action of a ligand. Negative modulation of receptor activity is achieved by phencyclidine (PCP) and magnesium ions.

Dizocilpine (MK-801) is the prototype compound in this class and has demonstrated efficacy in a number of animal models of focal ischaemia.[92-96] Unfortunately, a variety of safety concerns (including neuronal vacuolisation at relatively low doses) have stopped further development of this drug.[97]

Dextrorphan and dextromethorphan are both noncompetitive antagonists of the NMDA receptor at the phencyclidine binding site. In animal models, both have produced reductions in infarct volumes with administration either pre- or post-occlusion.[98-101] In humans, intravenous dextrorphan has significant adverse effects which limit its use (hallucinations, agitation, sedation, gastrointestinal disturbance and hypotension at high doses),[102] and its development has been ceased. Conversely, oral dextromethorphan (in dosages of 240 or 360mg daily for 3 weeks) does not cause any significant adverse effects.[103,104] Trials of this drug are ongoing.

Aptiganel (CNS-1102) has been shown to reduce infarct volumes, as well as the size of the ischaemic lesion on DWI, in rats after permanent middle cerebral artery occlusion (MCAO).[105-107] Clinical dose finding and tolerability studies with this compound showed a trend towards efficacy and did not identify any significant tolerability problems.[108] However, pivotal tolerability and efficacy studies have recently been suspended because of safety concerns, and final results are pending.

Pretreatment with remacemide, an anticonvulsant, prior to MCAO in a cat model has been shown to reduce the volume of ischaemic damage.[109] Preliminary results from a phase II safety and tolerability study in which patients were administered the drug within 12 hours of stroke onset demonstrated that the drug is well tolerated, but efficacy data have yet to be reported.[110,111]

Magnesium acts as an endogenous noncompetitive antagonist of the NMDA receptor, blocking the open channel in a voltage-dependent fashion.[112] *In vitro* and *in vivo* models of focal and global ischaemia have demonstrated that the ion possesses neuroprotective properties.[113-117] Muir and Lees[118] reported a placebo-controlled pilot trial involving 60 patients treated with intravenous magnesium within 12 hours after stroke onset. They showed a nonsignificant decrease in the number of early deaths in the magnesium-treated group, with no adverse effects. A larger multicentre trial [Intravenous Magnesium Efficacy in Stroke Trial (IMAGES)] is in progress.

Glutamate Binding Site Antagonists

A number of compounds compete with glutamate for its binding site on the NMDA receptor.

Selfotel (CGS-19755) was shown to attenuate neuronal degeneration and death in a number of animal models of diffuse or focal brain ischaemia, with neuroprotection conferred with administration up to 4 hours after the onset of ischaemia.[119-123] Efficacy in animal models and tolerability in phase II clinical trials[124,125] led to two almost identical large phase III clinical trials of a single intravenous dose of selfotel versus placebo administered within 6 hours of the onset of acute hemispheric infarction. However, these studies were terminated prematurely as a result of a statistically nonsignificant trend towards increased mortality in the active treatment group, and a low probability that efficacy would be demonstrated if the trial was continued.[126,127] A high incidence of adverse effects (affecting >50% of actively treated patients), especially neuropsychiatric effects (agitation, confusion, paranoia, delirium and hallucinations), were noted in the clinical studies and certainly would have complicated clinical use of this drug.

In animal models of cerebral ischaemia, treatment with other glutamate binding site blockers, such as D-CPPENE and CGP-40116, reduces infarct volumes.[128,129] There is, as yet, no data available on the effects of these drugs in humans.

Glycine Binding Site Antagonists

Glycine site antagonists have received less attention than other types of NMDA receptor antagonists. However, they have fewer adverse effects and, as a result, interest in them is increasing.

Kynurenic and thiokynurenic acid derivatives (such as 7-Cl kynurenate), HA-966 derivatives (such as L-687,414), derivatives of quinoxaline-2,3-dione (QX) [such as licostinel (ACEA-1021), ACEA-1031, and ZD-9379] and felbamate all downregulate the NMDA current by binding to the glycine site of the receptor. These drugs have been shown to have neuroprotective effects in animal models.[130-134] Some of these agents are not specific for the glycine site, since they also block AMPA or kainate receptors or possess the ability to lower body temperature or inhibit lipid peroxidation; properties which may contribute to their neuroprotective effect. Only a small number of these agents have been tested in humans. Data from clinical trials with licostinel and gavestinel (GV-150526A) show that these drugs are well tolerated by patients who have experienced a stroke.[135,136]

The anticonvulsant felbamate blocks sodium channels as well as the glycine binding site. In animal models, felbamate reduces ischaemic damage whether administered prior to or following the induction of ischaemia.[137,138] A worrying incidence of aplastic anaemia and hepatotoxicity with long term therapy led to the withdrawal of this drug from the market. The relevance of these adverse events to acute stroke therapy is unknown.

Polyamine Binding Site Antagonists

The endogenous polyamines spermine, spermidine and putrescine potentiate ion channel current in some subtypes of the NMDA receptor. The polyamine binding site of the NMDA receptor may be blocked with ifenprodil or eliprodil (SL-82.0715). In addition to blockade of the polyamine site, these drugs also block some VGCCs, reduce K^+-induced glutamate release and bind to sigma receptors.[139-141] These drugs have demonstrated neuroprotective effects in animal models.[142] Eliprodil has been investigated in clinical trials although the results have not been published. However, we believe further development of this compound has been discontinued.

Redox Binding Site

The redox state of the NMDA receptor modulates the amplitude of the channel current. In the oxidised state, sulphydryl groups of the channel protein can form disulphide bonds thus limiting the ion current. In the reduced state (the likely state in ischaemia), formation of free thiol (-SH) groups is favoured and the ion current increases. Oxidising agents or compounds which react with the free thiol groups can therefore limit the current and potentially be neuroprotective.[143]

Nitroglycerine (glyceryl trinitrate) and sodium nitroprusside have demonstrated some neuroprotective efficacy in animal models,[144,145] although drug-induced hypotension required correction. These drugs may act by transferring nitrosonium ion (NO^+) to the thiol groups of the NMDA receptor; however, their effect may also be mediated via nitric oxide–induced cerebral vasodilatation.

3.2.2 α-Amino-3-Hydroxy-5-Methyl-4-Isoxazole Propionic Acid Receptor Antagonists

A number of quinoxalinedione compounds are competitive AMPA receptor antagonists and have been assessed in animal models of ischaemia. Initially developed compounds were non-selective, also possessing NMDA antagonist properties through interaction with the glycine binding site; however, NCC-079202 (NBQX) proved to be selective for AMPA receptors.[146] While this compound demonstrated neuroprotective properties in animal models, dose related respiratory depression and nephrotoxicity (related to its poor solubility in aqueous solution) prevented its development for clinical use.[147-149]

The 2,3-benzodiazepine GYKI-52466 is a noncompetitive AMPA antagonist that has been shown to reduce infarct size in rat models of focal ischaemia.[149,150] However, the drug appears to have a very short therapeutic window, with administration only 2 hours after the induction of ischaemia being ineffective.[150,151]

LY-293558 is a competitive AMPA antagonist which is more soluble than either NCC-079202 or GYKI-52466, and has demonstrated neuroprotective effects in animal models.[152] However, this effect is not striking, perhaps because the compound is a competitive rather than a noncompetitive AMPA antagonist.

3.2.3 Metabotropic Receptor Ligands

Eight subtypes of metabotropic receptors have been identified and these can be divided into 3 groups on the basis of sequence homology and function.[17] Activation of group I receptors by excessive glutamate release triggers phosphoinositide hydrolysis (as described in section 1). Group II and, perhaps, group III receptors appear to have a role in limiting excitotoxic damage, as they are concentrated on presynaptic membranes where their activation inhibits neurotransmitter release. Specific agonists of group II receptors have been shown to protect neurons against hypoxia and toxicity mediated by stimulation of NMDA receptors *in vitro*.[153,154] The mixed nonselective glutamate receptor agonist ACPD, which preferentially activates group II receptors, was shown to reduce infarct volume by about one-third in a mouse model of focal ischaemia.[155] A number of specific group II receptor agonists (such as (+)LY 354740, DCG-IV) are currently being evaluated.

3.3 Inhibitors of Glutamate Release

The principal mechanisms by which drugs can inhibit glutamate release are sodium channel blockade, adenosine (A_1) receptor activation, or presynaptic calcium channel (N-, P- or Q-type) blockade.

3.3.1 Sodium Channel Antagonists

Anticonvulsants

The anticonvulsants phenytoin and its water-soluble derivative fosphenytoin, and lamotrigine and the related compounds BW-1003C87 and sipatrigine (BW-619C89) are all sodium channel antagonists which have cytoprotective properties.

Phenytoin and fosphenytoin have both demonstrated neuroprotective potential in animal models of cerebral ischaemia.[156-158] A multicentre placebo-controlled clinical study of fosphenytoin in acute ischaemic stroke is in progress.

Lamotrigine administered immediately after permanent MCAO in rats reduces total and cortical infarct volumes.[159] BW-1003C87 also protects against both global and focal ischaemia in rats.[160] However, the clinical use of this drug is limited by the fact that is inhibits dihydrofolate reductase, which could cause anaemia, thrombocytopenia and teratogenicity. Sipatrigine, a structural analogue of BW-1003C87, is devoid of antifolate activity and reduces infarct size in models of global and focal ischaemia.[161-163] When administered after MCAO, sipatrigine produced up to a 60% reduction in total infarct size, which was more evident in cortical than striatal regions.[162] Dose-related behavioural adverse effects were observed, but were generally minor. A dose-finding phase IIa trial of sipatrigine in acute ischaemic stroke has been completed; results showed that the drug was well tolerated.[164] Phase III trials are planned.

Lubeluzole

Lubeluzole is a benzothiazole derivative whose mechanisms of action include sodium channel blockade, inhibition of glutamate release and inhibition of nitric oxide–mediated toxicity. In a phase II trial, 193 patients were randomised within 6 hours of acute ischaemic stroke to receive lubeluzole 7.5mg over 1 hour followed by 10 mg/day for 5 days, lubeluzole 15mg over 1 hour followed by 20 mg/day for 5 days, or placebo.[165] The trial was terminated prematurely because of an imbalance in mortality between the groups. Mortality rates at 28 days for placebo, lubeluzole 10 mg/day and lubeluzole 20 mg/day were 18, 6 and 35%, respectively. Encouragingly, intravenous administration of lubeluzole 7.5mg over 1 hour followed by 10 mg/day was well tolerated and produced a statistically significant reduction in mortality.

Two pivotal phase III studies have been completed in North America and Europe/Australia.[166,167] A total of almost 1400 patients were randomised within 6 hours of stroke onset to receive either lubeluzole (7.5mg IV over 1 hour followed by continuous IV infusion of 10 mg/day for 5 days) or placebo. In the North American study,[166] a nonsignificant improvement in mortality and a significant improvement in measures of neurological recovery were observed at 12 weeks with lubeluzole treatment. In the European/Australian study,[167] the overall mortality rate at 3 months was similar for the lubeluzole and placebo treated groups. On post-hoc amalysis, stroke severity was found to be a determinant of treatment benefit. A clinically significant reduction in mortality was noted in the lubeluzole-treated patients for whom stroke severity was mild to moderate, but not in those with severe deficits. No tolerabilty concerns were seen with lubeluzole treatment. Despite these encouraging rsults, further developmemt of this drug has apparently been discontinued.

Lifarizine

Lifarizine, which possesses both sodium and calcium channel modulating properties, has been shown to be neuroprotective in both global and focal ischaemia models.[168-170] A pilot study in humans who were treated within 12 hours after stroke showed a trend towards improved outcomes in the lifarizine-treated patients.[171] However, lifarizine treatment produced falls in blood pressure, especially in elderly women in who a trend towards poorer outcomes, was observed. Further trials have been abandoned.

3.3.2 Adenosine Receptor Agonists

With ischaemia, the extracellular level of adenosine increases. This effect is thought to confer endogenous neuroprotection by activation of adenosine A_1 receptors which inhibit Ca^{++} influx, through P- and N-type VGCCs, and the release of neurotransmitters. Animal studies with A_1 receptor agonists, such as cyclohexyladenosine (CHA), have shown a significant reduction in neuronal death in models of global and focal ischaemia.[172-174] However, these drugs would be difficult to use clinically because of potent cardiovascular effects, including hypotension and cardiodepression.

A_2 receptors are involved in the regulation of CBF (mediating hypoxia-induced increases in CBF)[175] and neurotransmitter release, and activation of these receptors enhances ischaemic damage. Thus, acute therapy with A_2 receptor antagonists is neuroprotective.[176] Likewise, short term administration of A_1 receptor antagonists increases ischaemic damage; however, long term therapy is neuroprotective, perhaps because of an upregulation of A_1 receptors.[177]

3.4 Free Radical Scavengers

A number of compounds with free radical scavenging properties have been studied with the hope that they will negate the toxic effects of free radical species.

3.4.1 Tirilazad

Tirilazad (U-74006F) is a 21-aminosteroid (lazaroid), a derivative of methylprednisolone that is devoid of glucocorticoid properties. It is a potent scavenger of oxygen free radicals and inhibits lipid peroxidation.[178] It also attenuates the postischaemic elevation in leukotriene C_4 levels (probably by preventing lipid peroxide activation of 5-lipoxygenase),[179] reduces postischaemic cerebral hypoperfusion,[180] reduces cerebral oedema induced by MCAO,[181] and ameliorates impairment of cerebral metabolism in acidotic ischaemia.[182]

Phase II clinical trials showed that this drug in dosages up to 6.0 mg/kg/day was well tolerated by patients who had experienced a stroke.[183] A large scale (n = 414) tolerability and efficacy trial of tirilazad (6 mg/kg/day) administered within 6 hours of acute stroke onset was terminated after no statistically significant difference in functional outcome was found in active-treated compared with placebo-treated patients.[184] A further trial involving 556 patients who had experienced strokes and were treated with tirilazad (6 mg/kg/day for 3 days) within 6 hours of onset also found no improvement in overall functional outcome with therapy.[185] Development of this drug for stroke has been discontinued.

3.4.2 Nitrone-Based Free Radical Traps

Nitrones react with free radicals to form stable nitroxides. Nitrone-based free radical traps such as phenyl-t-butyl-nitrone (PBN) have been tested in animal models of focal and global ischaemia and demonstrated reduced ischaemic damage.[186-188] As yet, there have been no studies of these compounds in humans.

3.5 Opioid Receptor Antagonists

3.5.1 Naloxone

The opioid receptor antagonist naloxone has been found to reduce histological damage and neurological deficit after focal or global ischaemia in animal models.[189] However, after pilot clinical studies with this agent showed no beneficial effects,[190,191] no further studies have been performed for this indication.

3.5.2 Nalmefene

Nalmefene, an exomethylene derivative of naltrexone, is a selective antagonist of opioid κ-receptors that has a relatively long biological half-life. Nalmefene improved recovery of ischaemic brain tissue in animal models.[192,193] Recent work indicates that nalmefene inhibits glutamate release.[192] Nalmefene is now in phase II clinical trials for neuroprotection in stroke.[194]

3.6 Gangliosides

Gangliosides are sialic acid–containing glycosphingolipids found in the outer leaflet of the neuronal membrane lipid bilayer. They appear to play a role in signalling in neuronal membranes, and in nerve repair and regrowth.[195]

3.6.1 GM1 (Siagoside)

A purified preparation of monosialoganglioside (GM1; siagoside) has demonstrated neuroprotective effects in models of ischaemia. Possible mechanisms for this effect include inhibition of ischaemia-induced amino acid release,[196-199] inhibition of PLC and PLA_2 activation,[198] inhibition of NOS by binding calmodulin,[200] and, through its high affinity for Ca^{++}, reduction of transmembrane Ca^{++} influx.[201]

In early trials of the drug in patients who had experienced stroke,[202-204] purified bovine GM1 (40mg daily as intramuscular injections for 6 weeks) was compared with placebo. A significant improvement in outcome and an absence of adverse effects with GM1 treatment were reported. An Italian study of GM1 (100 mg/day intravenously) demonstrated a greater degree of early neurological improvement in GM1-treated patients than in placebo-treated patients, but the differences were not significant after 4 months.[205]

However, in two large trials, the Sygen Acute Stroke Study (SASS)[206] and the Early Stroke Trial (EST),[207] discouraging results were reported. In the SASS trial, 287 patients were randomised within 48 hours of stroke to either GM1 100mg intramuscularly or placebo for 28 days. No significant difference was found in mortality or overall functional outcome between the groups; however, motor function was significantly better at day 28 ($p < 0.02$) and approached significance at final follow-up (12 weeks; $p = 0.057$) in GM1-treated patients. In EST, 805 patients were randomised within 5 hours of stroke onset to GM1 (an initial intravenous dose of 200mg; a second dose of 100mg 12 hours later; a daily dose of 100mg intravenously from day 2 to 10 and intramuscularly from day 11 to 21) or placebo. Improvement in neurological status measured with the Canadian Neurological Score was greater in the GM1-treated group ($p = 0.06$). Post-hoc analysis showed significant improvement in neurological outcome at 4 months ($p = 0.016$) for patients treated within 4 hours after stroke onset.

Common adverse events associated with gangliosides include fever, rash, abnormal liver function, hypertension and seizures. Reports of acute axonal demyelinating polyneuropathy, complicating the parenteral use of ganglioside preparations, has discouraged their further development as long term stroke therapy.[207-211]

3.7 Growth Factors

It is believed that acidic and basic fibroblast growth factors (aFGF, bFGF), insulin-like growth factors I and II (IGF-I, IGF-II), ciliary neurotrophic factor (CNTF) and epidermal growth factor (EGF) all play a role in maturation, maintenance and repair of the nervous system. Increased levels of these factors and their receptors can be detected after ischaemia of brief duration in animals.[212-217] As a result, they have been investigated for neuroprotective efficacy in cerebral ischaemia.

The most extensively studied growth factor is bFGF, which has been demonstrated to reduce ischaemic neuronal loss in animal models.[218-221] Human trials with bFGF have been initiated. A North American study has recently been terminated because of tolerability concerns. A European/Australian study, using a slightly different treatment protocol, is ongoing.

Animal studies with aFGF, EGF and CNTF have all shown neuroprotection to varying degrees. The mechanisms by which these growth factors are neuroprotective are unknown, but possibilities include limiting the increase in intracellular Ca^{++} level, normalising the PKC phosphorylating system, and inhibiting nitric oxide–induced toxicity and oxidative damage.[222-224]

3.8 Antagonists of Inflammatory Cytokines

Increased expression of a number of inflammatory cytokines including interleukin (IL)-1β, IL-6 and tumour necrosis factor (TNF)α has been documented soon after the onset of cerebral ischaemia.[225-227] Of these cytokines, IL-1 is the best studied in cerebral ischaemia, although other cytokines, in particular IL-6 and TNFα, have also demonstrated neuroprotective properties in *in vitro* studies.[228,229]

3.8.1 Interleukin-1

IL-1 appears to play an important role in mediating aspects of ischaemic brain damage.[230] Antagonism of the effects of IL-1 can be achieved with IL-1 receptor antagonist (IL-1ra). This naturally occurring competitive antagonist of IL-1 has been shown to be neuroprotective in animal models of cerebral ischaemia.[231,232]. IL-1ra has a theoretical advantage over other neuroprotective agents in that it does not affect normal brain functioning (unlike, for example, NMDA receptor antagonists), as it is not involved in normal brain functioning but is specifically induced in response to injury.

3.9 Inhibitors of Cellular Adhesion

Leucocyte adhesion and activation at sites of cerebral ischaemia potentiates ischaemic neuronal damage by obstruction of the microvasculature and generation of toxic substances such as free radicals, granular enzymes and cytokines. Vascular endothelium usually exhibits low adhesiveness for leucocytes; however, when stimulated (e.g. by cytokines), surface adhesion molecules responsible for adhesion and activation of leucocytes are expressed by endothelial at sites of tissue damage. The intercellular adhesion molecule-1 (ICAM-1) is one of the immunoglobulin-type adhesion molecules expressed on the surface of activated endothelial cells.

Rats administered anti–ICAM-1 antibody immediately upon reperfusion after 2 hours of MCAO demonstrated a significant reduction in lesion volume, a reduction in neutrophil numbers in the ischaemic tissue and improved physiological function.[233] Further work indicated that the beneficial effect of anti–ICAM-1 antibody was seen after transient, but not permanent, MCAO.[234] This and that transient MCAO may predispose to the reperfusion injury associated with leucocyte adhesion suggests that anti–ICAM-1 antibody may be most beneficial when used with thrombolysis.[235]

Enlimomab is a murine monoclonal antibody specific for the second domain of human ICAM-1. A double-blind, randomised, clinical trial enroling 625 patients who received either enlimomab or placebo within 6 hours of ischaemic stroke has recently finished.[236] However, no significant improvements in outcome (measured using the Rankin scale, Barthel index or NIH Stroke scale) or patient survival were observed.

3.10 Other Agents

3.10.1 Potassium Channel Openers

Potassium channel openers act to reduce membrane excitability and stimulus-coupled neurotransmitter release from presynaptic terminals. Both these effects protect against ischaemic excitotoxicity by inhibition of presynaptic glutamate release and by postsynaptic hyperpolarisation, strengthening the voltage-dependent Mg^{++} blockade of the NMDA receptor and reducing Ca^{++} flux through VGCCs. These drugs may also be beneficial by causing cerebral vasodilatation through their actions on vascular smooth muscle. In animal studies, one of these compounds (Y26763) has been shown to reduce infarct volumes in a rat model.[237]

3.10.2 γ-Aminobutyric Acid Agonists

GABA receptor agonists might be expected to exert some neuroprotective effect by hyperpolarising the postsynaptic neuron and ameliorating the effects of excessive glutamatergic excitation. GABAergic agonists, such as diazepam or chlomethiazole, and inhibitors of GABA uptake such as vigabatrin have been shown to be neuroprotective in animal models.[238-245] Human trials with chlomethiazole have been conducted. Unpublished Phase III data from the Chlomethiazole Acute Stroke Study, in which 1360 patients were randomised to chlomethiazole (75 mg/kg intravenously over 24 hours) or placebo within 12 hours of stroke onset,[246,247] showed no significant benefit of treatment.

3.10.3 Nitric Oxide Synthase Inhibitors

NOS inhibitors might be neuroprotective by inhibiting the effects of nNOS and iNOS, but might also be harmful by inhibiting eNOS. NOS inhibitors which selectively reduce nNOS but not eNOS activity consistently demonstrate a neuroprotective effect in animal models.[248,249] Aminoguanidine, a relatively selective iNOS inhibitor, is similarly efficacious in animal models.[250]

3.10.4 Xanthine Oxidase Inhibitors

Xanthine oxidase inhibitors, including tocopherol (vitamin E), allopurinol, oxypurinol and MDL-74,180, have been tested for neuroprotective efficacy in animal models. They have been shown to reduce neuronal loss in global ischaemia and to reduce infarct size in focal ischaemia models.[251-255] These agents may have a role as adjuvant therapies in acute stroke.

3.10.5 Phospholipase C Inhibitors

The PLC inhibitor phenylmethylsulfonylfluoride has been tested in an animal model of global ischaemia but was not found to reduce neuronal loss.[256]

3.10.6 Calpain Inhibitors

Calpain inhibitors, such as CX295, Cbz-Val-Phe-H and calpain inhibitor I, have demonstrated neuroprotective efficacy in animal models of focal and global ischaemia.[257-259]

3.10.7 Cyclooxygenase and Lipoxygenase Inhibitors

Arachidonic acid, primarily produced by degradation of membrane phospholipids, may contribute to neuronal death: (i) directly through enhancement of NMDA receptor currents or the blockade of inhibitory transmission; or (ii) indirectly via its metabolites, thromboxanes and prostaglandins (produced via the cyclooxygenase pathway) and leukotrienes, lipoxins, hepoxillins and hydroxyeicosatetraenoic acid (HETE) [produced via the lipoxygenase pathway].

Cyclooxygenase inhibitors, such as aspirin, indomethacin and ibuprofen, have been evaluated in various animal models, but their neuroprotective effect is equivocal.[260,261] The established use of aspirin in the prevention of stroke would be enhanced by proof of a neuroprotective effect. While it is suggested that aspirin enhances the capacity of the brain to resist oxidative damage by free radicals,[262] this cytoprotective effect has not been formally tested in the clinical setting. However, a recent retrospective analysis failed to detect any difference in stroke severity between patients taking aspirin at the time of their stroke and those who were not.[263] Similarly, in both IST[58] and CAST,[61] there was no demonstrated treatment effect, apart from a reduction in the risk of early stroke recurrence.

Lipoxygenase inhibitors, such as docebenone (AA-861), mixed cyclooxygenase-lipoxygenase inhibitors, such as BW-755C, and compounds which also inhibit PLA_2, such as EPC-K1 and LY-178002, have been tested in animals and produced reductions in ischaemic damage.[264-267]

3.10.8 Citicoline

Citicoline (cytidine-5-diphosphocholine; CDP-choline) is a precursor of the cell membrane component phosphatidylcholine. Hydrolysis of phosphatidylcholine during ischaemia to yield free fatty acids, which may in turn generate free radical species, can be reversed by exogenous administration of citicoline.[268] Citicoline has been shown to be beneficial in animal models of ischaemia and hypoxia.[269-271]

In a phase II clinical trial, 272 patients with moderate-to-severe acute cerebral infarction, who were admitted within 14 days of the ictus, were randomised to receive either citicoline (1g intravenously daily for 14 days) or placebo. The patients treated with citicoline showed significant improvements in level of consciousness compared with the placebo-treated patients, and the drug seemed well tolerated.[272] In a recent US trial, 259 patients were randomised within 24 hours of stroke onset to one of 3 dosages of citicoline (500mg, 1g or 2g per day for 6 weeks) or placebo. A significant difference in functional and neurological outcomes measured with Barthel and Rankin indices, National Institutes of Health Stroke Scale (NIHSS) and the Mini-Mental State Examination (MMSE) was observed in favour of citicoline treatment with 500mg of citicoline emerging as the optimal dose.[273] Further phase III evaluation is ongoing.

3.10.9 Piracetam

Piracetam, a GABA derivative, is a so-called nootropic drug (a drug that affects intellectual functioning). It has been used to improve memory and learning and appears to act by facilitating cholinergic and excitatory amine neurotransmission.[274] It also increases the fluidity of neuronal membranes and possesses haemorheological properties, increasing red cell deformability and decreasing platelet aggregation.

Pilot studies in humans suggested a beneficial effect when given early after acute stroke and these led to the Piracetam in Acute Stroke Study (PASS). Patients were randomised to either piracetam (a 12g intravenous bolus followed by 12g daily for 4 weeks and 4.8g daily for 8 weeks) or placebo within 12 hours after stroke onset. Piracetam treatment produced no difference in mortality, neurological deficit or functional disability compared with placebo.[275] Post-hoc subgroup analysis of patients randomised within 7 hours of onset showed a trend towards improved neurological function, and a significant decrease in functional disability with piracetam treatment, especially in patients with moderate-to-severe stroke. Further studies with this agent looking at treatment within 7 hours of stroke are planned.

3.10.10 Ebselen

Ebselen is a lipid-soluble, seleno-organic compound which potently inhibits lipid peroxidation through a glutathione peroxidase–like action. In a recent study, in which 300 patients were randomised within 48 hours of ischaemic stroke to either ebselen or placebo, ebselen-treated patients had a significantly better outcome, especially if treated within 24 hours of onset.[276]

3.10.11 Allosteric Modifiers of Haemoglobin

Allosteric modifiers of haemoglobin increase oxygen delivery to the tissues by shifting the haemoglobin-oxygen dissociation curve in a similar way to 2,3-diphosphoglycerate (2,3-DPG). RSR-13 given intravenously prior to permanent MCAO in a cat model reduced infarct size.[277] Efficacy with treatment delayed until after the onset of ischaemia is yet to be established. A theoretical problem with this form of therapy may be increased generation of oxygen free radicals; however, the reduction in infarct volumes in this study suggests this may not be a practical problem.

3.10.12 Apoptosis Inhibitors

Inhibition of apoptosis may be another way of limiting cell death after ischaemia.[30] The gene Bcl-2 and proteolytic enzymes such as the caspases have been shown to play an important role in apoptotic cell death in other cell types, and their role in apoptotic neuronal death is being investigated. A neuroprotective effect of Bcl-2 has been shown in transgenic animals that overexpress Bcl-2, and in models of focal or global ischaemia when viral vectors are used to overexpress Bcl-2.[278-281]

Caspase inhibitors, such as z-VAD-DCB, YVAD-chloromethyl-ketone and DEVD-fluoromethyl-ketone, are also reported to be neuroprotective in focal cerebral ischaemia models when administered intraventricularly.[282,283]

4. Conclusion

A large number of drugs with varying mechanisms of action have been studied in humans, but, as yet, there is no clearly effective, universally applicable treatment for acute ischaemic stroke. Of the treatments outlined in sections 2 and 3, thrombolysis with alteplase has shown the most promise as an effective acute treatment in clinical trials. However, it is currently an option only for a select group of patients who experience a stroke (i.e. those presenting to hospital within the first 3 hours after stroke onset) and it still carries a risk of adverse outcome from haemorrhagic transformation. None of the currently available neuroprotective agents have demonstrated unequivocal efficacy when administered after stroke in humans, although a number of compounds are in development.

Given the complexity of the ischaemic cascade, it is possible that a cocktail of drugs, with differing mechanisms of action, may be necessary to effectively ameliorate ischaemic damage after stroke. Combinations of neuroprotective agents,[284-287] as well as combining neuroprotection with thrombolysis,[288-294] have been studied in animals with encouraging results, but, as yet, have not been subjected to clinical trials. Neuroprotective agents administered early may act synergistically with thrombolysis, and may also prolong the therapeutic window for thrombolysis, thus increasing the number of stroke patients who may benefit from that therapy. Logically, the next step is to combine neuroprotection with thrombolysis in clinical trials.

It is of some concern that so many potential therapies have shown promise in animal models only to fail on human testing. Fundamental differences between the animal models used to test these drugs and human stroke are likely to underpin these failures. In particular, the homogenous nature of animal models, where variables such as the duration and severity of the ischaemic insult can be closely controlled, contrast markedly with the heterogeneity of mechanism and severity inherent in humans who experience stroke.

As stroke is such a heterogeneous disorder, it is possible that a drug has already been tested that is effective in a subgroup of patients who have experienced stroke but which is of no benefit or is harmful in others, thus resulting in negative results when tested in unselected patients. Some studies of neuroprotective agents performed thus far have shown benefits to subsets of patients on post-hoc analysis (e.g. lubeluzole, citicoline and piracetam).[166,167,273,275] To identify an effective treatment for stroke, it may be necessary to conduct trials which compare subsets of patients who have experienced strokes. Perhaps advances in neuroimaging, such as DWI and perfusion MRI, may assist in selecting patients for inclusion in trials and provide more homogeneous study populations.

Acknowledgements

Dr Read is supported by a scholarship from the National Health and Medical Research Council of Australia.

References

1. Astrup J, Siesjo BK, Symon L. Thresholds in cerebral ischaemia: the ischaemic penumbra. Stroke 1981; 12: 723-5
2. Astrup J, Symon L, Branston NM, et al. Cortical evoked potential and extracellular K^+ and H^+ at critical levels of brain ischaemia. Stroke 1977; 8: 51-7
3. Jones TH, Morawetz RB, Crowell RM, et al. Thresholds of focal cerebral ischaemia in awake monkeys. J Neurosurg 1981; 54: 773-82
4. Wise RJS, Bernardi S, Frackowiak RSJ, et al. Serial observations on the pathophysiology of acute stroke: the transition from ischaemia to infarction as reflected in regional oxygen extraction. Brain 1983; 106: 197-222
5. Heiss W-D, Huber M, Fink GR, et al. Progressive derangement of periinfarct viable tissue in ischaemic stroke. J Cereb Blood Flow Metab 1992; 12: 193-203
6. Marchal G, Beaudouin V, Rioux P, et al. Prolonged persistence of substantial volumes of potentially viable brain tissue after stroke: a correlative PET-CT study with voxel-based data analysis. Stroke 1996; 27: 599-606
7. Furlan M, Marchal G, Viader F, et al. Spontaneous neurological recovery after stroke and the fate of the ischaemic penumbra. Ann Neurol 1996; 40: 216-26
8. Kohno K, Hoehn-Berlage M, Mies G, et al. Relationship between diffusion-weighted MR images, cerebral blood flow, and energy state in experimental brain infarction. Magn Reson Imaging 1995; 13: 73-80
9. Harris RJ, Symon L, Branston NM, et al. Changes in extracellular calcium activity in cerebral ischaemia. J Cereb Blood Flow Metab 1981; 1: 203-9
10. Harris RJ, Symon L. Extracellular pH, potassium and calcium activities in progressive ischaemia of rat cortex. J Cereb Blood Flow Metab 1984; 4: 178-86
11. Shimada N, Graf R, Rosner G, et al. Ischaemic flow threshold for extracellular glutamate increase in cat cortex. J Cereb Blood Flow Metab 1989; 9: 603-6
12. Shimada N, Graf R, Rosner G, et al. Differences in ischaemia-induced accumulation of amino acids in the cat cortex. Stroke 1990; 21: 1445-51
13. Matsumoto K, Graf R, Rosner G, et al. Elevation of neuroactive substances in the cortex of cats during prolonged focal ischaemia. J Cereb Blood Flow Metab 1993; 13: 586-94
14. Choi DW. Excitotoxic cell death. J Neurobiol 1992; 23: 1261-76
15. Miller RJ. Multiple calcium channels and neuronal function. Science 1987; 235: 46-52
16. Siesjo BK. Pathophysiology and treatment of focal cerebral ischaemia: pt II: mechanisms of damage and treatment. J Neurosurg 1992; 77: 337-54
17. Pin JP, Duvoisin R. Neurotransmitter receptors I. the metabotropic glutamate receptors: structure and functions. Neuropharmacology 1995; 34: 1-26
18. Katsura K, Rodriguez de Turco EB, Folbergrova J, et al. Coupling among energy failure, loss of ion homeostasis, and phospholipase A2 and C activation during ischaemia. J Neurochem 1993; 61: 1677-84
19. Miller B, Sarantis M, Traynelis SF, et al. Potentiation of NMDA receptor currents by arachidonic acid. Nature 1992; 355: 722-5

20. Schwartz RD, Yu X. Inhibition of GABA-gated chloride channel function by arachidonic acid. Brain Res 1992; 585: 405-10
21. Chen L, Huang LY. Protein kinase C reduces Mg2+ block of NMDA-receptor channels as a mechanism of modulation. Nature 1992; 356: 521-3
22. Siman R, Noszek JC. Excitatory amino acids activate calpain I and induce structural protein breakdown *in vivo*. Neuron 1988; 1: 279-87
23. Gunter TE, Pfeiffer DR. Mechanisms by which mitochondria transport calcium. Am J Physiol 1990; 258: C755-86
24. Zoratti M, Szabo I. The mitochondrial permeability transition. Biochim Biophys Acta 1995; 1241: 139-76
25. Moncada S, Higgs A. The L-arginine-nitric oxide pathway. N Engl J Med 1993; 329: 2002-12
26. Samdani AF, Dawson TM, Dawson VL. Nitric oxide synthase in models of focal ischaemia. Stroke 1997; 28: 1283-8
27. Radi R, Beckman JS, Bush KM, et al. Peroxynitrite-induced membrane lipid peroxidation: the cytotoxic potential of superoxide and nitric oxide. Arch Biochem Biophys 1991; 288: 481-7
28. Dawson TM, Snyder SH. Gases as biological messengers: nitric oxide and carbon monoxide in the brain. J Neurosci 1994; 14: 5147-59
29. del Zoppo GJ. Microvascular changes during cerebral ischaemia and reperfusion. Cerebrovasc Brain Metab Rev 1994; 6: 47-96
30. MacManus JP, Linnik MD. Gene expression induced by cerebral ischaemia: an apoptotic perspective. J Cereb Blood Flow Metab 1997; 17: 815-32
31. del Zoppo GJ. Thrombolytic therapy in cerebrovascular disease. Stroke 1988; 19: 1174-9
32. von Kummer R, Hacke W. Safety and efficacy of intravenous tissue plasminogen activator and heparin in acute middle cerebral artery stroke. Stroke 1992; 23: 646-52
33. Brott TG, Haley EC Jr, Levy DE, et al. Urgent therapy for stroke. Pt I. pilot study of tissue plasminogen activator administered within 90 minutes. Stroke 1992; 23: 632-40
34. Haley EC Jr, Levy DE, Brott TG, et al. Urgent therapy for stroke: pt II. pilot study of tissue plasminogen activator administered 91-180 minutes from onset. Stroke 1992; 23: 641-5
35. Haley EC Jr, Brott TG, Sheppard GL, et al. The t-PA Bridging Study Group. Pilot randomised trial of tissue plasminogen activator in acute ischaemic stroke. Stroke 1993; 24: 1000-4
36. Yamaguchi T, Hayakawa T, Kiuchi H, et al. Intravenous tissue plasminogen activator ameliorates the outcome of hyperacute embolic stroke. Cerebrovasc Dis 1993; 3: 269-72
37. Hommel M, Cornu C, Boutitie F, et al. Thrombolytic therapy with streptokinase in acute ischaemic stroke. N Engl J Med 1996; 335: 145-50
38. Donnan GA, Davis SM, Chambers BR, et al. For the Australian Streptokinase (ASK) Trial Study Group. Streptokinase for acute ischaemic stroke with relationship to time of administration. JAMA 1996; 276: 961-6
39. Multicentre Acute Stroke Trial - Italy (MAST-I) Group. Randomised controlled trial of streptokinase, aspirin, and combination of both in treatment of acute ischaemic stroke. Lancet 1995; 346: 1509-14
40. Hacke W, Kaste M, Fieschi C, et al. For the European Cooepartive Acute Stroke Study (ECASS). Intravenous thrombolysis with recombinant tissue plasminogen activator for acute hemispheric stroke. JAMA 1995; 274: 1017-25
41. The National Institute of Neurological Disorders and Stroke rt-PA Stroke Study Group. Tissue plasminogen activator for acute ischaemic stroke. N Engl J Med 1995; 333: 1581-7
42. Wardlaw JM, Warlow CP, Counsell C. Systematic review of evidence on thrombolytic therapy for acute ischaemic stroke. Lancet 1997; 350: 607-14
43. Morris AD, Ritchie C, Grosset DG, et al. A pilot study of streptokinase for acute cerebral infarction. Q J Med 1995; 88: 727-31
44. Mori E, Yoneda Y, Tabuchi M, et al. Intravenous recombinant tissue plasminogen activator in acute carotid artery territory stroke. Neurology 1992; 42: 976-82
45. Abe T, Kazama M, Naito I, et al. Clinical evaluation for efficacy of tissue cultured urokinase (TCUK) on cerebral thrombosis by means of multi-centre double blind study. Blood Vessels 1981; 12: 321-41
46. Ohtomo E, Araki G, Itoh E, et al. Clinical efficacy of urokinase in the treatment of cerebral thrombosis: multi-centre double blind study in comparison with placebo. Clin Eval 1985; 15: 711-31
47. Atarashi I, Ohtomo E, Araki G et al. Clincal utility of urokinase in the treatment of acute stage cerebral thrombosis: multi-centre double blind study in comparison with placebo. Clin Eval 1985; 13: 659-709
48. Yamaguchi T. Japanese Thrombolysis Study Group. Intravenous tissue plasminogen activator in acute thromboembolic stroke: a placebo controlled, double blind trial. In: del Zoppo GJ, Mori E, Hacke W, editors. Thrombolytic therapy in acute ischaemic stroke II. New York: Springer Verlag, 1993: 59-65
49. Hacke W, Kaste M, Fieschi C, et al. Randomised double-blind placebo-controlled trial of thrombolytic therapy with intravenous altepase in acute ischaemic stroke (ECASS II). Lancet 1998; 352: 1245-51
50. del Zoppo GJ, Ferbert A, Otis S, et al. Local intra-arterial fibrinolytic therapy in acute carotid territory stroke: a pilot study. Stroke 1988; 19: 307-13
51. Mori E, Tabuchi M, Yoshida T, et al. Intracarotid urokinase with thromboembolic occlusion of the middle cerebral artery. Stroke 1988; 19: 801-12
52. Hacke W, Zeumer H, Ferbert A, et al. Intra-arterial thrombolytic therapy improves outcome in patients with acute vertebrobasilar occlusive disease. Stroke 1988; 19: 1216-22
53. del Zoppo GJ, Higashida RT, Furlan AJ, et al. PROACT: a phase II randomized trial of recombinant pro-urokinase by direct arterial delivery in acute middle cerebral artery stroke. Stroke 1998; 29: 4-11

54. Howard AW, Aaron SD. Low molecular weight heparin decreases proximal and distal deep venous thrombosis following total knee arthroplasty: a meta-analysis of randomized trials. Thromb Haemost 1998; 79: 902-6
55. Palmer AJ, Koppenhagen K, Kirchhof B, et al. Efficacy and safety of low molecular weight heparin, unfractionated heparin and warfarin for thrombo-embolism prophylaxis in orthopaedic surgery: a meta-analysis of randomised clinical trials. Haemostasis 1997; 27: 75-84
56. Palmer AJ, Schramm W, Kirchhof B, et al. Low molecular weight heparin and unfractionated heparin for prevention of thrombo-embolism in general surgery: a meta-analysis of randomised clinical trials. Haemostasis 1997; 27; 65-74
57. Turpie AG. Prophylaxis of venous thromboembolism in stroke patients. Semin Thromb Hemost 1997; 23: 155-7
58. International Stroke Trial Collaborative Group. The International Stroke Trial (IST): a randomised trial of aspirin, subcutaneous heparin, both, or neither among 19,435 patients with acute ischaemic stroke. Lancet 1997; 349: 1569-81
59. Kay R, Wong KS, Yu YL, et al. Low-molecular-weight heparin for the treatment of acute ischaemic stroke. N Engl J Med 1995; 333: 1588-93
60. The Publications Committee for the Trial of ORG 10172 in Acute Stroke Treatment (TOAST) Investigators. Low molecular weight heparinoid, ORG 10172 (Danaparoid), and outcome after acute ischaemic stroke: a randomised controlled trial. JAMA 1988; 279: 1265-72
61. CAST (Chinese Acute Stroke Trial) Collaborative Group. CAST: randomised placebo-controlled trial of early aspirin use in 20,000 patients with acute ischaemic stroke. Lancet 1997; 349: 1641-9
62. Allen GS, Ahn HS, Preziosi TJ, et al. Cerebral arterial spasm: a controlled trial of nimodipine in patients with subarachnoid haemorrhage. N Engl J Med 1983; 308: 619-24
63. Petruk KC, West M, Mohr G, et al. Nimodipine treatment in poor-grade aneurysm patients: results of a multicenter double-blind placebo-controlled trial. J Neurosurg 1988; 68: 505-17
64. Öhman J, Heiskanen O. Effect of nimodipine on the outcome of patients after aneurysmal subarachnoid haemorrhage and surgery. J Neurosurg 1988; 69: 683-6
65. Jan M, Buchheit F, Tremoulet M. Therapeutic trial of intravenous nimodipine in patients with established cerebral vasospasm after rupture of intracranial aneurysms. Neurosurgery 1988; 23: 154-7
66. Pickard JD, Murray GD, Illingworth R, et al. Effect of oral nimodipine on cerebral infarction and outcome after subarachnoid haemorrhage: British aneurysm nimodipine trial. BMJ 1989; 298: 636-42
67. Milde LN, Milde JH, Michenfelder JD. Delayed treatment with nimodipine improves cerebral blood flow after complete cerebral ischaemia in the dog. J Cereb Blood Flow Metab 1986; 6: 332-7
68. Gotoh O, Mohamed AA, McCulloch J, et al. Nimodipine and histopathological consequences of middle cerebral artery occlusion in the rat. J Cereb Blood Flow Metab 1986; 6: 321-31
69. Steen PA, Newberg LA, Milde JM, et al. Nimodipine improves cerebral blood flow and neurologic recovery after complete ischaemia in the dog. J Cereb Blood Flow Metab 1983; 3: 38-43
70. Steen PA, Gisvold SE, Milde JH, et al. Nimodipine improves outcome when given after complete cerebral ischaemia in primates. Anesthesiology 1985; 62: 406-14
71. Gelmers HJ, Gorter K, de Weerdt CJ, et al. A controlled trial of nimodipine in acute ischaemic stroke. N Engl J Med 1988; 318: 203-7
72. Bogousslavsky J, Regli F, Zumstein V, et al. Double-blind study of nimodipine in non-severe stroke. Eur Neurol 1990; 30: 23-6
73. Martínez-Vila E, Guillén F, Villanueva JA, et al. Placebo-controlled trial of nimodipine in the treatment of acute ischaemic cerebral infarction. Stroke 1990; 21: 1023-8
74. TRUST Study Group. Randomised, double-blind, placebo-controlled trial of nimodipine in acute stroke. Lancet 1990; 336: 1205-9
75. The American Nimodipine Study Group. Clinical trial of nimodipine in acute ischaemic stroke. Stroke 1992; 23: 3-8
76. Krämer G, Tettenborn B, Schmutzhard E, et al. Nimodipine in acute ischaemic stroke: results of the Nimodipine German-Austrian Stroke Trial. Cerebrovasc Dis 1994; 4: 182-8
77. Hennerici M, Krämer G, North PM, et al. Nimodipine in the treatment of acute MCA ischaemic stroke. Cerebrovasc Dis 1994; 4: 189-93
78. Kaste M, Fogelholm R, Erilä T, et al. A randomized, double-blind, placebo-controlled trial of nimodipine in acute ischaemic hemispheric stroke. Stroke 1994; 25: 1348-53
79. Mohr JP, Orgogozo JM, Harrison MJG, et al. Meta-analysis of oral nimodipine trials in acute ischaemic stroke. Cerebrovasc Dis 1994; 4: 197-203
80. Limburg M. Very early nimodipine use in stroke - the first 100 patients: cooperation between GPs and neurologists [abstract]. Stroke 1996; 27: 172
81. Norris JW, LeBrun LH, Anderson BA, et al. Intravenous nimodipine in acute ischaemic stroke. Cerebrovasc Dis 1994; 4: 194-6
82. Bridgers SL, Koch G, Munera C, et al. Intravenous nimodipine in acute stroke: interim analysis of randomized trials [abstract]. Stroke 1991; 22: 153
83. Wahlgren NG, MacMahon DG, De Keyser J, et al. For the INWEST Study Group. Intravenous Nimodipine West European Stroke Trial (INWEST) of nimodipine in the treatment of acute ischaemic stroke. Cerebrovasc Dis 1994; 4: 204-10
84. Azcona A, Lataste X. Isradipine in patients with acute ischaemic cerebral infarction: an overview of the ASCLEPIOS programme. Drugs 1990; 40 Suppl. 2: 52-7
85. Lataste X, Maurer W, Whitehead J et al. Application of sequential methods to clinical trial in stroke: the ASCLEPIOS study. 2nd World Congress of Stroke: 1992 SEP 8-12; Washington DC, S16

86. Oczkowski WJ, Hachinski V, Bogousslavsky J, et al. A double-blind, randomised trial of PY 108-068 in acute ischaemic cerebral infarction. Stroke 1989; 20: 604-8
87. Limburg M, Hijdra A. Flunarizine in acute ischaemic stroke: a pilot study. Eur Neurol 1990; 30: 121-2
88. Prange H, Hartung J, Hertel G, et al. For the German Flunarizine Group. Treatment of acute stroke with flunarizine IV. International Cönference on Stroke; 1991: Geneva, Switzerland, 39
89. Takizawa S, Matsushima K, Fujita H, et al. A selective N-type calcium channel antagonist reduces extracellular glutamate release and infarct volume in focal cerebral ischaemia. J Cereb Blood Flow Metab 1995; 15: 611-8
90. Yenari MA, Palmer JT, Sun GH, et al. Time-course and treatment response with SNX-111, an N-type calcium channel blocker, in a rodent model of focal cerebral ischaemia using diffusion-weighted MRI. Brain Res 1996; 739: 36-45
91. Bowersox SS, Singh T, Luther RR. Selective blockade of N-type voltage-sensitive calcium channels protects against brain injury after transient cerebral ischaemia in rats. Brain Res 1997; 747: 343-7
92. Kochhar A, Zivin JA, Lyden PD, et al. Glutamate antagonist therapy reduces neurologic deficits produced by focal central nervous system ischaemia. Arch Neurol 1988; 45: 148-53
93. Ozyurt E, Graham DI, Woodruff GN, et al. Protective effect of the glutamate antagonist, MK-801, in focal cerebral ischaemia in the cat. J Cereb Blood Flow Metab 1988; 8: 138-43
94. Park CK, Nehls DG, Graham DI, et al. Focal cerebral ischaemia in the cat: treatment with the glutamate antagonist MK-801 after induction of ischaemia. J Cereb Blood Flow Metab 1988; 8: 757-62
95. Park CK, Nehls DG, Graham DI, et al. The glutamate antagonist MK-801 reduces focal ischaemic damage in the rat. Ann Neurol 1988; 24: 543-51
96. Park CK, Nehls DG, Teasdale GM, et al. Effect of the NMDA antagonist MK-801 on local cerebral blood flow in focal cerebral ischaemia in the rat. J Cereb Blood Flow Metab 1989; 9: 617-2
97. Olney JW, Labruyere J, Price MT. Pathological changes induced in cerebrocortical neurons by phencyclidine and related drugs. Science 1989; 244: 1360-2
98. George CP, Goldberg MP, Choi DW, et al. Dextromethorphan reduces neocortical ischaemic neuronal damage *in vivo*. Brain Res 1988; 440: 375-9
99. Steinberg GK, George CP, DeLaPaz R, et al. Dextromethorphan protects against cerebral injury following transient focal ischaemia in rabbits. Stroke 1988; 19: 1112-8
100. Steinberg GK, Saleh J, Kunis D. Delayed treatment with dextromethorphan and dextrorphan reduces cerebral damage after transient focal ischaemia. Neurosci Lett 1988; 89: 193-7
101. Steinberg GK, Saleh J, Kunis D, et al. Protective effect of N-methyl-D-aspartate antagonist after focal ischaemia in rabbits. Stroke 1989; 20: 1247-52
102. Albers GW, Atkinson RP, Kelley RE, et al. Safety, tolerability and pharmacokinetics of the N-methyl-D-aspartate antagonist dextrorphan in patients with acute stroke. Stroke 1995; 26: 254-8
103. Albers GW, Saenz RE, Moses JA Jr, et al. Safety and tolerance of oral dextromethorphan in patients at risk for brain ischaemia. Stroke 1991; 22: 1075-7
104. Albers GW, Saenz RE, Moses JA Jr. Tolerability of oral dextromethorphan in patients with a history of brain ischaemia. Clin Neuropharmacol 1992; 15: 509-14
105. Minematsu K, Fisher M, Li L, et al. Effects of a novel NMDA antagonist on experimental stroke rapidly and quantitatively assessed by diffusion-weighted MRI. Neurology 1993; 43: 397-403
106. Minematsu K, Fisher M, Li L, et al. Diffusion and perfusion magnetic resonance imaging studies to evaluate a noncompetitive N-methyl-D-aspartate antagonist and reperfusion in experimental stroke in rats. Stroke 1993; 24: 2074-81
107. Meadows M-E, Fisher M, Minematsu K. Delayed treatment with a noncompetitive NMDA antagonist, CNS-1102, reduces infarct size in rats. Cerebrovasc Dis 1994; 4: 26-31
108. Fisher M. For CNS 1102-003 Investigators. Cerestat (CNS 1102), a non-competitive NMDA antagonist, in ischaemic stroke patients: dose-escalating safety study [abstract]. Cerebrovasc Dis 1994; 4: 245
109. Bannan PE, Graham DI, Lees KR, et al. Neuroprotective effect of remacemide hydrochloride in focal cerebral ischaemia in the cat. Brain Res 1994; 664: 271-5
110. Muir KW, Lees KR. Initial experience with remacemide hydrochloride in patients with acute ischaemic stroke. Ann N Y Acad Sci 1995; 765: 322-3
111. Dyker AG, Muir KW, Lees KR. A double-blind, randomised, placebo controlled, dose-escalation study of remacemide in patients with acute stroke [abstract]. Stroke 1997; 28: 233
112. Nowak L, Bregestovski P, Ascher P, et al. Magnesium gates glutamate-activated channels in mouse central neurones. Nature 1984; 307: 462-5
113. Finkbeiner S, Stevens CF. Applications of quantitative measurements for assessing glutamate neurotoxicity. Proc Natl Acad Sci U S A 1988; 85: 4071-4
114. Stys PK, Ransom BR, Waxman SG. Effects of polyvalent cations and dihydropyridine calcium channel blockers on recovery of CNS white matter from anoxia. Neurosci Lett 1990; 115: 293-9
115. McDonald JW, Silverstein FS, Johnston MV. Magnesium reduces N-methyl-D-aspartate (NMDA)-mediated brain injury in perinatal rats. Neurosci Lett 1990; 109: 234-8
116. Tsuda T, Kogure K, Nishioka K, et al. Mg2+ administered up to twenty-four hours following reperfusion prevents ischaemic damage of the CA1 neurons in the rat hippocampus. Neuroscience 1991; 44: 335-41
117. Izumi Y, Roussel S, Pinard E, et al. Reduction of infarct volume by magnesium after middle cerebral artery occlusion in rats. J Cereb Blood Flow Metab 1991; 11: 1025-30

118. Muir KW, Lees KR. A randomized, double-blind, placebo-controlled pilot trial of intravenous magnesium sulfate in acute stroke. Stroke 1995; 26: 1183-8
119. Pérez-Pinzón MA, Maier CM, Yoon EJ, et al. Correlation of CGS 19755 neuroprotection against *in vitro* excitotoxicity and focal cerebral ischaemia. J Cereb Blood Flow Metab 1995; 15: 865-76
120. Takizawa S, Hogan M, Hakim AM. The effects of a competitive NMDA receptor antagonist (CGS-19755) on cerebral blood flow and pH in focal ischaemia. J Cereb Blood Flow Metab 1991; 11: 786-93
121. Grotta JC, Picone CM, Ostrow PT, et al. CGS-19755, a competitive NMDA receptor antagonist, reduces calcium-calmodulin binding and improves outcome after global cerebral ischaemia. Ann Neurol 1990; 27: 612-9
122. Swan JH, Meldrum BS. Protection by NMDA antagonists against selective cell loss following transient ischaemia. J Cereb Blood Flow Metab 1990; 10: 343-51
123. Simon R, Shiraishi K. N-methyl-D-aspartate antagonist reduces stroke size and regional glucose metabolism. Ann Neurol 1990; 27: 606-11
124. Clark WM, Coull BM, CGS 19755 Study Group. Randomized trial of CGS 19755, a glutamate antagonist, in acute ischaemic stroke treatment. Neurology 1994; 44 Suppl. 2: A270
125. Grotta J, Clark W, Coull B, et al. Safety and tolerability of the glutamate antagonist CGS 19755 (Selfotel) in patients with acute ischaemic stroke: results of a phase IIa randomized trial. Stroke 1995; 26: 602-5
126. Davis SM. For the ASSIST Collaborative Group. Acute stroke studies involving selfotel treatment (ASSIST) [abstract]. Stroke 1997; 28: 271
127. Davis SM, Albers GW, Diener H-C, et al. Termination of acute stroke studies involving selfotel treatment [letter]. Lancet 1997; 349: 32
128. Park CK, McCulloch J, Kang JK, et al. Pretreatment with a competitive NMDA antagonist D-CPPene attenuates focal cerebral infarction and brain swelling in awake rats. Acta Neurochir 1994; 127; 220-6
129. Sauer D, Weber E, Luond G, et al. The competitive NMDA antagonist CGP 40116 permanently reduces brain damage after middle cerebral artery occlusion in rats. J Cereb Blood Flow Metab 1995; 15: 602-10
130. Moroni F, Alesiani M, Facci L, et al. Thiokynurenates prevent excitotoxic neuronal death *in vitro* and *in vivo* by acting as glycine antagonists and as inhibitors of lipid peroxidation. Eur J Pharmacol 1992; 218: 145-51
131. Gill R, Hargreaves RJ, Kemp JA. The neuroprotective effect of the glycine site antagonist 3R-(+)-cis-4-methyl-HA966 (L-687,414) in a rat model of focal ischaemia. J Cereb Blood Flow Metab 1995; 15: 197-204
132. Warner DS, Martin H, Ludwig P, et al. *In vivo* models of cerebral ischaemia: effects of parenterally administered NMDA receptor glycine site antagonists. J Cereb Blood Flow Metab 1995; 15: 188-96
133. Takano K, Tatlisumak T, Formato JE, et al. Glycine site antagonist attenuates infarct size in experimental focal ischaemia: postmortem and diffusion mapping studies. Stroke 1997; 28: 1255-63
134. Pietra C, Ziviani L, Valerio E, et al. Neuroprotection by GV150526A: comparison with reference compounds [abstract]. Stroke 1996; 27: 189
135. Albers GW, Clark WM, Atkinson RP, et al. Dose escalation study of the NMDA glycine-site antagonist ACEA 1021 in acute ischaemic stroke [abstract]. Stroke 1997; 28: 233
136. Dyker AG, Lees KR, Preston C, et al. The safety, tolerability and pharmacokinetics of GV150526A in patients with acute stroke [abstract]. Stroke 1997; 28: 233
137. Wasterlain CG, Adams LM, Schwartz PH, et al. Posthypoxic treatment with felbamate is neuroprotective in a rat model of hypoxia-ischaemia. Neurology 1993; 43: 2303-10
138. Wasterlain CG, Adams LM, Hattori H, et al. Felbamate reduces hypoxic-ischaemic brain damage *in vivo*. Eur J Pharmacol 1992; 212: 275-8
139. Church J, Fletcher EJ, Baxter K, et al. Blockade by ifenprodil of high voltage-activated Ca2+ channels in rat and mouse cultured hippocampal pyramidal neurones: comparison with N-methyl-D-aspartate receptor antagonist actions. Br J Pharmacol 1994; 113: 499-507
140. Contreras PC, Bremer ME, Gray NM. Ifenprodil and SL 82.0715 potently inhibit binding of [3H] (+)-3-PPP to sigma binding sites in rat brain. Neurosci Lett 1990; 116: 190-3
141. Karbon EW, Patch RJ, Pontecorvo MJ, et al. Ifenprodil potently interacts with [3H] (+)-3-PPP-labeled sigma binding sites in guinea pig brain membranes. Eur J Pharmacol 1990; 176: 247-8
142. Gotti B, Duverger D, Bertin J, et al. Ifenprodil and SL 82.0715 as cerebral anti-ischaemic agents: I. evidence for efficacy in models of cerebral ischaemia. J Pharmacol Exp Ther 1988; 247: 1211-21
143. Stamler JS, Singel DJ, Loscalzo J. Biochemistry of nitric oxide and its redox-activated forms. Science 1992; 258; 1898-902
144. Zhang F, Iadecola C. Nitroprusside improves blood flow and reduces brain damage after focal ischaemia. Neuroreport 1993; 4: 559-62
145. Sathi S, Edgecomb P, Warach S, et al. Chronic transdermal niroglycerine (NTG) is neuroprotective in experimental rodent stroke models. Soc Neurosci Abst 1993; 19: 849
146. Sheardown MJ, Nielsen EO, Hansen AJ, et al. 2,3-Dihydroxy-6-nitro-7-sulfamoyl-benzo(F)quinoxaline: a neuroprotectant for cerebral ischaemia. Science 1990; 247: 571-4
147. Buchan AM, Xue D, Huang ZG, et al. Delayed AMPA receptor blockade reduces cerebral infarction induced by focal ischaemia. Neuroreport 1991; 2: 473-6
148. Gill R, Nordholm L, Lodge D. The neuroprotective actions of 2,3-dihydroxy-6-nitro-7-sulfamoyl-benzo(F)quinoxaline (NBQX) in a rat focal ischaemia model. Brain Res 1992; 580: 35-43
149. Xue D, Huang ZG, Barnes K, et al. Delayed treatment with AMPA, but not NMDA, antagonists reduces neocortical infarction. J Cereb Blood Flow Metab 1994; 14: 251-61

150. Smith SE, Meldrum BS. Cerebroprotective effect of a non-N-methyl-D-aspartate antagonist, GYKI 52466, after focal ischaemia in the rat. Stroke 1992; 23: 861-4
151. Le Peillet E, Arvin B, Moncada C, et al. The non-NMDA antagonists, NBQX and GYKI 52466, protect against cortical and striatal cell loss following transient global ischaemia in the rat. Brain Res 1992; 571: 115-20
152. Bullock R, Graham DI, Swanson S, et al. Neuroprotective effect of the AMPA receptor antagonist LY-293558 in focal cerebral ischaemia in the cat. J Cereb Blood Flow Metab 1994; 14: 466-71
153. Bruno V, Battaglia G, Copani A, et al. Activation of class II or III metabotropic glutamate receptors protects cultured cortical neurons against excitotoxic degeneration. Eur J Neurosci 1995; 7: 1906-13
154. Buisson A, Yu SP, Choi DW. DCG-IV selectively attenuates rapidly triggered NMDA-induced neurotoxicity in cortical neurons. Eur J Neurosci 1996; 8: 138-43
155. Chiamulera C, Albertini P, Valerio E, et al. Activation of metabotropic receptors has a neuroprotective effect in a rodent model of focal ischaemia. Eur J Pharmacol 1992; 216: 335-6
156. Boxer PA, Cordon JJ, Mann ME, et al. Comparison of phenytoin with noncompetitive N-methyl-D-aspartate antagonists in a model of focal brain ischaemia in rat. Stroke 1990; 21 Suppl. 3: 47-51
157. Rataud J, Debarnot F, Mary V, et al. Comparative study of voltage-sensitive sodium channel blockers in focal ischaemia and electric convulsions in rodents. Neurosci Lett 1994; 172: 19-23
158. Urenjak J, Obrenovitch TP. Pharmacological modulation of voltage-gated Na+ channels: a rational and effective strategy against ischaemic brain damage. Pharmacol Rev 1996; 48: 21-67
159. Smith SE, Meldrum BS. Cerebroprotective effect of lamotrigine after focal ischaemia in rats. Stroke 1995; 26: 117-22
160. Meldrum BS, Swan JH, Leach MJ, et al. Reduction of glutamate release and protection against ischaemic brain damage by BW1003C87. Brain Res 1992; 593: 1-6
161. Graham SH, Chen J, Lan J, et al. Neuroprotective effects of a use-dependent blocker of voltage-dependent sodium channels, BW619C89, in rat middle cerebral artery occlusion. J Pharmacol Exp Ther 1994; 269: 854-9
162. Leach MJ, Swan JH, Eisenthal D, et al. BW619C89, a glutamate release inhibitor, protects against focal cerebral ischaemic damage. Stroke 1993; 24: 1063-7
163. Smith SE, Lekieffre D, Sowinski P, et al. Cerebroprotective effect of BW619C89 after focal or global cerebral ischaemia in the rat. Neuroreport 1993; 4: 1339-42
164. Hussein Z, Fraser IJ, Lees KR, et al. Pharmacokinetics of 619C89, a novel neuronal sodium channel inhibitor, in acute stroke patients after loading and discrete maintenance infusions. Br J Clin Pharmacol 1996; 41: 505-11
165. Diener HC, Hacke W, Hennerici M, et al. For the Lubeluzole International Study Group. Lubeluzole in acute ischaemic stroke: a double-blind, placebo-controlled phase II trial. Stroke 1996; 27: 76-81
166. Grotta J. For the US and Canadian Lubeluzole Ischaemic Stroke Study Group. Lubeluzole treatment of acute ischaemic stroke. Stroke 1997; 28: 2338-46
167. Diener HC. European and Australian Lubeluzole Ischaemic Stroke Study Group. Multinational randomised controlled trial of lubeluzole in acute ischaemic stroke. Cerebrovasc Dis 1998; 8: 172-81
168. Brown CM, Calder C, Linton C, et al. Neuroprotective properties of lifarizine compared with those of other agents in a mouse model of focal cerebral ischaemia. Br J Pharmacol 1995; 115: 1425-32
169. McBean DE, Winters V, Wilson AD, et al. Neuroprotective efficacy of lifarizine (RS-87476) in a simplified rat survival model of 2 vessel occlusion. Br J Pharmacol 1995; 116: 3093-8
170. Alps BJ, Calder C, Wilson AD, et al. Reduction by lifarizine of the neuronal damage induced by cerebral ischaemia in rodents. Br J Pharmacol 1995; 115: 1439-46
171. Squire IB, Lees KR, Pryse-Phillips W, et al. The effects of lifarizine in acute cerebral infarction: a pilot safety study. Cerebrovasc Dis 1996; 6: 156-60
172. von Lubitz DK, Dambrosia JM, Kempski O, et al. Cyclohexyl adenosine protects against neuronal death following ischaemia in the CA1 region of the gerbil hippocampus. Stroke 1988; 19: 1133-9
173. Januszewicz von Lubitz DK, Dambrosia JM, Redmond DJ. Protective effect of cyclohexyl adenosine in treatment of cerebral ischaemia in gerbils. Neuroscience 1989; 30: 451-62
174. Zhou JG, Meno JR, Hsu SS, et al. Effects of theophylline and cyclohexyladenosine on brain injury following normo- and hyperglycemic ischaemia: a histopathologic study in the rat. J Cereb Blood Flow Metab 1994; 14: 166-73
175. Phillis JW. Adenosine in the control of the cerebral circulation. Cerebrovasc Brain Metab Rev 1989; 1: 26-54
176. von Lubitz DK, Lin RCS, Jacobson KA. Cerebral ischaemia in gerbils: effects of acute and chronic treatment with adenosine A2A receptor agonist and antagonist. Eur J Pharmacol 1995; 287: 295-302
177. Rudolphi KA, Schubert P, Parkinson FE, et al. Adenosine and brain ischaemia. Cerebrovasc Brain Metab Rev 1992; 4: 346-69
178. Braughler JM, Hall ED, Jacobsen EJ, et al. The 21-amino-steroids: potent inhibitors of lipid peroxidation for the treatment of central nervous system trauma and ischaemia. Drugs Future 1989; 14: 143-52
179. Andrus PK, Taylor BM, Sun FF, et al. Effects of the lipid peroxidation inhibitor tirilazad mesylate (U-74006F) on gerbil brain eicosanoid levels following ischaemia and reperfusion. Brain Res 1994; 659: 126-32
180. Hall ED, Yonkers PA. Attenuation of postischemic cerebral hypoperfusion by the 21-aminosteroid U74006F. Stroke 1988; 19: 340-4
181. Young W, Wojak JC, DeCrescito V. 21-aminosteroid reduces ion shifts and edema in the rat middle cerebral artery occlusion model of regional ischaemia. Stroke 1988; 19: 1013-9
182. Kim H, Koehler RC, Hurn PD, et al. Amelioration of impaired cerebral metabolism after severe acidotic ischaemia by tirilazad posttreatment in dogs. Stroke 1996; 27: 114-21

183. The STIPAS Investigators. Safety study of tirilazad mesylate in patients with acute ischaemic stroke (STIPAS). Stroke 1994; 25: 418-23
184. Peters GR, Hwang L-J, Musch B, et al. Safety and efficacy of 6 mg/kg/day tirilazad mesylate in patients with acute ischaemic stroke (TESS study) [abstract]. Stroke 1996; 27: 195
185. The RANTTAS Investigators. A randomized trial of tirilazad mesylate in patients with acute stroke (RANTTAS). Stroke 1996; 27: 1453-8
186. Cao X, Phillis JW. α-phenyl-tert-butyl-nitrone reduces cortical infarct and edema in rats subjected to focal ischaemia. Brain Res 1994; 644: 267-72
187. Zhao Q, Pahlmark K, Smith ML, et al. Delayed treatment with the spin trap α-phenyl-tert-butyl nitrone (PBN) reduces infarct size following transient middle cerebral artery occlusion in rats. Acta Physiol Scand 1994; 152: 349-50
188. Yue TL, Gu JL, Lysko PG, et al. Neuroprotective effects of phenyl-t-butyl-nitrone in gerbil global brain ischaemia and in cultured rat cerebellar neurons. Brain Res 1992; 574: 193-7
189. Hosobuchi Y, Baskin DS, Woo SK. Reversal of induced ischaemic neurological deficit in gerbils by the opiate antagonist naloxone. Science 1982; 215: 69-71
190. Federico F, Lucivero V, Lamberti P, et al. A double blind randomized pilot trial of naloxone in the treatment of acute ischaemic stroke. Ital J Neurol Sci 1991; 12: 557-63
191. Olinger CP, Adams HP Jr, Brott TG, et al. High-dose intravenous naloxone for the treatment of acute ischaemic stroke. Stroke 1990; 21: 721-5
192. Faden AI, Shirane R, Chang LH, et al. Opiate-receptor antagonist improves metabolic recovery and limits neurochemical alterations associated with reperfusion after global brain ischemia in rats. J Pharmacol Exp Ther 1990; 255: 451-8
193. Yum SW, Faden AI. Comparison of the neuroprotective effects of the N-methyl-D-aspartate antagonist MK-801 and the opiate-receptor antagonist nalmefene in experimental spinal cord ischemia. Arch Neurol 1990; 47: 277-81
194. Clark WM, Ertag W, Orecchio EJ, et al. For the Cervene Stroke Study Investigators. Cervene in acute ischaemic stroke: results of a double-blind, placebo-controlled, dose-comparison study [abstract]. Stroke 1997; 28: 233
195. Carolei A, Fieschi C, Bruno R, et al. Monosialoganglioside GM1 in cerebral ischaemia. Cerebrovasc Brain Metab Rev 1991; 3: 134-57
196. Vaccarino F, Guidotti A, Costa E. Ganglioside inhibition of glutamate-mediated protein kinase C translocation in primary cultures of cerebellar neurons. Proc Natl Acad Sci U S A 1987; 84: 8707-11
197. Simon RP, Chen J, Graham SH. GM1 ganglioside treatment of focal ischaemia: a dose-response and microdialysis study. J Pharmacol Exp Ther 1993; 265: 24-9
198. Lombardi G, Moroni F. GM1 ganglioside reduces ischaemia-induced excitatory amino acid output: a microdialysis study in the gerbil hippocampus. Neurosci Lett 1992; 134: 171-4
199. Phillis JW, O'Regan MH. GM1 ganglioside inhibits ischaemic release of amino acid neurotransmitters from rat cortex. Neuroreport 1995; 6: 2010-2
200. Dawson TM, Hung K, Dawson VL, et al. Neuroprotective effects of gangliosides may involve inhibition of nitric oxide synthase. Ann Neurol 1995; 37: 115-8
201. Costa E, Armstrong DM, Guidotti A, et al. Gangliosides in the protection against glutamate toxicity. Prog Brain Res 1994; 101: 357-73
202. Bassi S, Albizzati MG, Sbacchi M, et al. Double-blind evaluation of monosialoganglioside (GM1) therapy in stroke. J Neurosci Res 1984; 12: 493-398
203. Battistin L, Cesari A, Galligioni F, et al. Effects of GM1 ganglioside in cerebrovascular diseases: a double-blind trial in 40 cases. Eur Neurol 1985; 24: 343-51
204. Hoffbrand BI, Bingley PJ, Oppenheimer SM, et al. Trial of ganglioside GM1 in acute stroke. J Neurol Neurosurg Psychiatry 1988; 51: 1213-4
205. Argentino C, Sacchetti ML, Toni D, et al. GM1 ganglioside therapy in acute ischaemic stroke. Stroke 1989; 20: 1143-9
206. Alter M for the SASS investigators. Ganglioside GM1 in acute ischaemic stroke: the SASS trial. Stroke 1994; 25: 1141-8
207. Lenzi GL, Grigoletto F, Gent M, et al. Early treatment of stroke with monosialoganglioside GM-1: efficacy and safety results of the early stroke trial. Stroke 1994; 25: 1552-8
208. Schönhöfer PS. Guillain-Barre syndrome and parenteral gangliosides [letter]. Lancet 1991; 338: 757
209. Figueras A, Morales-Olivas FJ, Capella D, et al. Bovine gangliosides and acute motor polyneuropathy. BMJ 1992; 305: 1330-1
210. Landi G, D'Alessandro RD, Dossi BC, et al. Guillain Barre syndrome after exogenous gangliosides in Italy. BMJ 1993; 307: 1463-4
211. Illa I, Ortiz N, Gallard E, et al. Acute axonal Guillain-Barre syndrome with IgG antibodies against motor axons following parenteral gangliosides. Ann Neurol 1995; 38: 218-24
212. Kiyota Y, Takami K, Iwane M, et al. Increase in basic fibroblast growth factor-like immunoreactivity in rat brain after forebrain ischaemia. Brain Res 1991; 545: 322-8
213. Takami K, Kiyota Y, Iwane M, et al. Upregulation of fibroblast growth factor-receptor messenger RNA expression in rat brain following transient forebrain ischaemia. Exp Brain Res 1993; 97: 185-94
214. Guan J, Williams C, Gunning M, et al. The effects of IGF-1 treatment after hypoxic-ischaemic brain injury in adult rats. J Cereb Blood Flow Metab 1993; 13: 609-16
215. Beilharz EJ, Bassett NS, Sirimanne ES, et al. Insulin-like growth factor II is induced during wound repair following hypoxic-ischaemic injury in the developing rat brain. Brain Res Mol Brain Res 1995; 29: 81-91

216. Bergstedt K, Wieloch T. Changes in insulin-like growth factor 1 receptor density after transient cerebral ischaemia in the rat: lack of protection against ischaemic brain damage following injection of insulin-like growth factor 1. J Cereb Blood Flow Metab 1993; 13: 895-8
217. Stephenson DT, Rash K, Clemens JA. Increase in insulin-like growth factor II receptor within ischaemic neurons following cerebral infarction. J Cereb Blood Flow Metab 1995; 15: 1022-31
218. Nakata N, Kato H, Kogure K. Protective effects of basic fibroblast growth factor against hippocampal neuronal damage following cerebral ischaemia in the gerbil. Brain Res 1993; 605: 354-6
219. Koketsu N, Berlove DJ, Moskowitz MA, et al. Pretreatment with intraventricular basic fibroblast growth factor decreases infarct size following focal cerebral ischaemia in rats. Ann Neurol 1994; 35: 451-7
220. Fisher M, Meadows ME, Do T, et al. Delayed treatment with intravenous basic fibroblast growth factor reduces infarct size following permanent focal cerebral ischaemia in rats. J Cereb Blood Flow Metab 1995; 15: 953-9
221. Tanaka R, Miyasaka Y, Yada K, et al. Basic fibroblast growth factor increases regional cerebral blood flow and reduces infarct size after experimental ischaemia in a rat model. Stroke 1995; 26: 2154-8
222. Mattson MP, Cheng B. Growth factors protect neurons against excitotoxic/ischaemic damage by stabilizing calcium homeostasis. Stroke 1993; 24 Suppl. 1: 136-40
223. Louis JC, Magal E, Gerdes W, et al. Survival-promoting and protein kinase C-regulating roles of basic FGF for hippocampal neurons exposed to phorbol ester, glutamate and ischaemia-like conditions. Eur J Neurosci 1993; 5: 1610-21
224. Maiese K, Boniece I, DeMeo D, et al. Peptide growth factors protect against ischaemia in culture by preventing nitric oxide toxicity. J Neurosci 1993; 13: 3034-40
225. Minami M, Kuraishi Y, Yabuuchi K, et al. Induction of interleukin-1β mRNA in rat brain after transient forebrain ischaemia. J Neurochem 1992; 58: 390-2
226. Wang X, Yue TL, Barone FC, et al. Concomitant cortical expression of TNFα and IL-1β mRNAs follows early response gene expression in transient focal ischaemia. Mol Chem Neuropathol 1994; 23: 103-14
227. Wang X, Yue TL, Young PR, et al. Expression of interleukin-6, c-fos, and zif268 mRNAs in rat ischaemic cortex. J Cereb Blood Flow Metab 1995; 15: 166-71
228. Yamada M, Hatanaka H. Interleukin-6 protects cultured rat hippocampal neurons against glutamate-induced cell death. Brain Res 1994; 643: 173-80
229. Cheng B, Christakos S, Mattson MP. Tumor necrosis factors protect neurons against metabolic-excitotoxic insults and promote maintenance of calcium homeostasis. Neuron 1994; 12: 139-53
230. Yamasaki Y, Matsuura N, Shozuhara H, et al. Interleukin-1 as a pathogenetic mediator of ischaemic brain damage in rats. Stroke 1995; 26: 676-80
231. Relton JK, Rothwell NJ. Interleukin-1 receptor antagonist inhibits ischaemic and excitotoxic neuronal damage in the rat. Brain Res Bull 1992; 29: 243-6
232. Loddick SA, Rothwell NJ. Neuroprotective effects of human recombinant interleukin-1 receptor antagonist in focal cerebral ischaemia in the rat. J Cereb Blood Flow Metab 1996; 16: 932-40
233. Zhang RL, Chopp M, Li Y, et al. Anti-ICAM-1 antibody reduces ischaemic cell damage after transient middle cerebral artery occlusion in the rat. Neurology 1994; 44: 1747-51
234. Zhang RL, Chopp M, Jiang N, et al. Anti-intercellular adhesion molecule-1 antibody reduces ischaemic cell damage after transient but not permanent middle cerebral artery occlusion in the Wistar rat. Stroke 1995; 26: 1438-42
235. Bowes MP, Zivin JA, Rothlein R. Monoclonal antibody to the ICAM-1 adhesion site reduces neurological damage in a rabbit cerebral embolism stroke model. Exp Neurol 1993; 119: 215-9
236. The Enlimomab Acute Stroke Trial Investigators. The Enlimomab acute stroke trial: final results. Cerebrovasc Dis 1997; 7 Suppl. 4: 18
237. Takaba H, Nagao T, Yao H, et al. An ATP-sensitive potassium channel activator reduces infarct volume in focal cerebral ischaemia in rats. Am J Physiol 1997; 2 Pt 2: R583-6
238. Johansen FF, Diemer NH. Enhancement of GABA neurotransmission after cerebral ischaemia in the rat reduces loss of hippocampal CA1 pyramidal cells. Acta Neurol Scand 1991; 84: 1-6
239. Voll CK, Auer RN. Postischemic seizures and necrotising ischaemic brain damage: neuroprotective effect of postischemic diazepam and insulin. Neurology 1991; 41: 423-8
240. Schwartz RD, Huff RA, Yu X, et al. Postischemic diazepam is neuroprotective in the gerbil hippocampus. Brain Res 1994; 647: 153-60
241. Schwartz RD, Yu X, Katzman MR, et al. Diazepam, given postischemia, protects selectively vulnerable neurons in the rat hippocampus and striatum. J Neurosci 1995; 15: 529-39
242. Abel MS, McCandless DW. Elevated γ-aminobutyric acid levels attenuate the metabolic response to bilateral ischaemia. J Neurochem 1992; 58: 740-4
243. Shuaib A, Ijaz S, Hasan S, et al. Gamma-vinyl GABA prevents hippocampal and substantia nigra reticulata damage in repetitive transient forebrain ischaemia. Brain Res 1992; 590: 13-7
244. Cross AJ, Jones JA, Baldwin HA, et al. Neuroprotective activity of chlomethiazole following transient forebrain ischaemia in the gerbil. Br J Pharmacol 1991; 104: 406-11
245. Snape MF, Baldwin HA, Cross AJ, et al. The effects of chlormethiazole and nimodipine on cortical infarct area after focal cerebral ischaemia in the rat. Neuroscience 1993; 53: 837-44
246. Wahlgren NG. For the Clomethiazole Acute Stroke Study Collaborative Group. The Clomethiazole Acute Stroke Study (CLASS): I: results of a randomised controlled study of clomethiazole versus placebo in 1360 acute stroke patients. Cerebrovasc Dis 1997; 7 Suppl. 4: 19

247. Wahlgren NG. For the Clomethiazole Acute Stroke Study Collaborative Group. The Clomethiazole Acute Stroke Study (CLASS): II: results of a randomised controlled study of clomethiazole versus placebo in 545 acute stroke patients classified as Total Anterior Circulation Syndrome (TACS). Cerebrovasc Dis 1997; 7 Suppl. 4: 19
248. Yoshida T, Limmroth V, Irikura K, et al. The NOS inhibitor, 7-nitroindazole, decreases focal infarct volume but not the response to topical acetylcholine in pial vessels. J Cereb Blood Flow Metab 1994; 14: 924-9
249. Zhang ZG, Reif D, Macdonald J, et al. ARL 17477, a potent and selective neuronal NOS inhibitor decreases infarct volume after transient middle cerebral artery occlusion in rats. J Cereb Blood Flow Metab 1996; 16: 599-604
250. Zhang F, Casey RM, Ross ME, et al. Aminoguanidine ameliorates and L-arginine worsens brain damage from intraluminal middle cerebral artery occlusion. Stroke 1996; 27: 317-23
251. Hara H, Kato H, Kogure K. Protective effect of α-tocopherol on ischaemic neuronal damage in the gerbil hippocampus. Brain Res 1990; 510: 335-8
252. Cowley DJ, Lukovic L, Petty MA. MDL 74,180 reduces cerebral infarction and free radical concentrations in rats subjected to ischaemia and reperfusion. Eur J Pharmacol 1996; 298: 227-33
253. Soloniuk DS, Perkins E, Wilson JR. Use of allopurinol and deferoxamine in cellular protection during ischaemia. Surg Neurol 1992; 38: 110-3
254. Lin Y, Phillis JW. Oxypurinol reduces focal ischaemic brain injury in the rat. Neurosci Lett 1991; 126: 187-90
255. Lin Y, Phillis JW. Deoxycoformycin and oxypurinol: protection against focal ischaemic brain injury in the rat. Brain Res 1992; 571: 272-80
256. Umemura A, Mabe H, Nagai H. A phospholipase C inhibitor ameliorates postischemic damage in rats. Stroke 1992; 23: 1163-6
257. Rami A, Krieglstein J. Protective effects of calpain inhibitiors against neuronal damage caused by cytotoxic hypoxia *in vitro* and ischaemia *in vivo*. Brain Res 1993; 609: 67-70
258. Hong SC, Goto Y, Lanzino G, et al. Neuroprotection with a calpain inhibitor in a model of focal cerebral ischaemia. Stroke 1994; 25: 663-9
259. Bartus RT, Hayward NJ, Elliott PJ, et al. Calpain inhibitor AK295 protects neurons from focal brain ischaemia: effects of postocclusion intra-arterial administration. Stroke 1994; 25: 2265-70
260. Johshita H, Asano T, Hanamura T, et al. Effect of indomethacin and a free radical scavenger on cerebral blood flow and edema after cerebral artery occlusion in cats. Stroke 1989; 20: 788-94
261. Cole DJ, Patel PM, Reynolds L, et al. Temporary focal cerebral ischaemia in spontaneously hypertensive rats: the effect of ibuprofen on infarct volume. J Pharmacol Exp Ther 1993; 266: 1713-7
262. Kuhn W, Muller T, Buttner T, et al. Aspirin as a free radical scavenger: consequences for therapy of cerebrovascular ischaemia. Stroke 1995; 26: 1959-60
263. Karepov V, Bornstein NM, Hass Y, et al. Does daily aspirin diminish severity of first-ever stroke? Arch Neurol 1997; 54: 1369-71
264. Namura Y, Shio H, Kimura J. LTC4/LTB4 alterations in rat forebrain ischaemia and reperfusion and effects of AA-861, CV-3988. Acta Neurochir 1994; 60 Suppl.: 296-9
265. Chen J, Weinstein PR, Graham SH. Attenuation of postischemic brain hypoperfusion and reperfusion injury by the cyclooxygenase-lipoxygenase inhibitor BW755C. J Neurosurg 1995; 83: 99-104
266. Block F, Kunkel M, Sontag K-H. Posttreatment with EPC-K1, an inhibitor of lipid peroxidation and of phospholipase A2 activity, reduces functional deficits after global ischaemia in rats. Brain Res Bull 1995; 36: 257-60
267. Clemens JA, Ho PPK, Panetta JA. LY178002 reduces rat brain damage after transient global forebrain ischaemia. Stroke 1991; 22: 1048-52
268. Trovarelli G, de Medio GE, Dorman RV, et al. Effect of cytidine diphosphate choline (CDP-choline) on ischaemia-induced alterations of brain lipid in the gerbil. Neurochem Res 1981; 6: 821-33
269. Kakihana M, Fukuda N, Suno M, et al. Effects of CDP-choline on neurologic deficits and cerebral glucose metabolism in a rat model of cerebral ischaemia. Stroke 1988; 19: 217-22
270. Dorman RV, Dabrowiecki Z, Horrocks LA. Effects of CDP- choline and CDP-ethanolamine on the alterations in rat brain lipid metabolism induced by global ischaemia. J Neurochem 1983; 40: 276-9
271. Yamamoto M, Shimizu M, Okamiya H. Pharmacological actions of a new TRH analogue, YM-14673, in rats subjected to cerebral ischaemia and anoxia. Eur J Pharmacol 1990; 181: 207-14
272. Tazaki Y, Sakai F, Otomo E, et al. Treatment of acute cerebral infarction with a choline precursor in a multicenter, double-blind, placebo-controlled study. Stroke 1988; 19: 211-6
273. Clark WM, Warach SJ, Pettigrew LC, et al. A randomised dose-response trial of citicoline in acute ischaemic stroke patients. Neurology 1997; 49: 671-8
274. Gouliaev AH, Senning A. Piracetam and other structurally related nootropics. Brain Res Brain Res Rev 1994; 19: 180-222
275. De Deyn P, De Reuck J, Vlietinck R, et al. Treatment of acute ischaemic stroke with piracetam. Stroke 1997; 28: 2347-52
276. Yamaguchi T, Sano K, Takakura K, et al. Ebselen in acute ischaemic stroke: a placebo-controlled, double-blind clinical trial. Stroke 1998; 29: 12-7
277. Watson JC, Doppenberg EM, Bullock MR, et al. Effects of the allosteric modification of hemoglobin on brain oxygen and infarct size in a feline model of stroke. Stroke 1997; 28: 1624-30
278. Choi DW. Ischaemia-induced neuronal apoptosis. Curr Opin Neurobiol 1996; 6: 667-72
279. Chopp M, Li Y. Apoptosis in focal cerebral ischaemia. Acta Neurochir Suppl (Wien) 1996; 66: 21-6
280. Linnik MD. Role of apoptosis in acute neurodegenerative disorders. Restorative Neurol Neurosci 1996; 9: 219-25

281. Lawrence MS, Ho DY, Sun GH, et al. Overexpression of Bcl-2 with herpes simplex vectors protects CNS neurons against neurological insults *in vitro* and *in vivo*. J Neurosci 1996; 16: 486-96
282. Loddick SA, MacKenzie A, Rothwell NJ. An ICE inhibitor, z-VAD-DCB attenuates ischaemic brain damage in the rat. Neuroreport 1996; 7: 1465-8
283. Hara H, Friedlander RM, Gagliardini V, et al. Inhibition of interleukin 1β converting enzyme family proteases reduces ischaemic and excitotoxic neuronal damage. Proc Natl Acad Sci U S A 1997; 94: 2007-12
284. Lyden PD, Lonzo L. Combination therapy protects ischaemic brain in rats: a glutamate antagonist plus a gamma-aminobutyric acid agonist. Stroke 1994; 25: 189-96
285. Lyden P, Lonzo L, Nunez S. Combination chemotherapy extends the therapeutic window to 60 minutes after stroke. J Neurotrauma 1995; 12: 223-30
286. Aronowski J, Strong R, Grotta JC. Combined neuroprotection and reperfusion therapy for stroke: effect of lubeluzole and diaspirin cross-linked hemoglobin in experimental focal ischaemia. Stroke 1996; 27: 1571-6
287. Uematsu D, Araki N, Greenberg J, et al. Combined therapy with MK-801 and nimodipine for protection of ischaemic brain damage. Neurology 1991; 41: 88-94
288. Meden P, Overgaard K, Sereghy T, et al. Enhancing the efficacy of thrombolysis by AMPA receptor blockade with NBQX in a rat embolic stroke model. J Neurol Sci 1993; 119: 209-16
289. Bednar MM, Raymond-Russell SJ, Booth CL, et al. Combination tissue plasminogen activator and ticlopidine therapy in a rabbit model of acute thromboembolic stroke. Neurol Res 1996; 18: 45-8
290. Lekieffre D, Benavides J, Scatton B, et al. Neuroprotection afforded by a combination of eliprodil and a thrombolytic agent, rt-PA, in a rat thromboembolic stroke model. Brain Res 1997; 776: 88-95
291. Sereghy T, Overgaard K, Boysen G. Neuroprotection by excitatory amino acid antagonist augments the benefit of thrombolysis in embolic stroke in rats. Stroke 1993; 24: 1702-8
292. Overgaard K, Sereghy T, Pedersen H, et al. Neuroprotection with NBQX and thrombolysis with rt-PA in rat embolic stroke. Neurol Res 1993; 15: 344-9
293. Zivin JA, Mazzarella V. Tissue plasminogen activator plus glutamate antagonist improves outcome after embolic stroke. Arch Neurol 1991; 48: 1235-8
294. Bowes M, Rothlein R, Fagan S, et al. Monoclonal antibodies preventing leukocyte activation reduce experimental neurologic injury and enhance efficacy of thrombolytic therapy. Neurology 1995; 45: 815-9

Correspondence: Prof. *Geoffrey A. Donnan*, Department of Neurology, Austin and Repatriation Medical Centre, Heidelberg, Victoria 3084, Australia.

Therapeutic Window in Ischaemic Stroke

Experimental Concepts, Neuroimaging Studies and Implications for Pharmacological Treatment

Wolf-Dieter Heiss and *Rudolf Graf*

Max-Planck-Institut für Neurologische Forschung and Neurologische Universitätsklinik, Cologne, Germany

Experimental studies in animal models and cell cultures have formed the basis of current concepts of the pathophysiology of ischaemic brain damage. Ischaemic cell death is hypothesised to be a consequence of progressive deleterious interactions between various circulatory, biochemical and molecular disturbances (for reviews, see Siesjö,[1] Pulsinelli,[2] and Kogure et al.[3]), which are all, in principle, amenable to therapeutic interventions.[4] The transfer of many biochemical, and most molecular, data from the experimental to the clinical setting is still limited. However, insight into the dynamics of the development of ischaemic damage has an impact on the management of acute stroke, e.g. for the selection of patients who might benefit from early reperfusion, as achieved by thrombolytic therapy.

For brain tissue to function it must have an adequate supply of blood. Consequently, damage will occur if there is an impairment of blood supply, with the severity and extent of permanent neurological defects being dependent on the amount of tissue suffering an impairment of blood supply below certain flow thresholds for critical time periods.

Experimental work on ischaemic flow thresholds has demonstrated the existence of two critical levels of decreased perfusion: (i) a level below which reversible neuronal failure occurs (functional threshold); and (ii) a lower threshold below which irreversible membrane failure and morphological damage occur (for a review see Heiss[5]) [fig. 1]. The range of perfusion values between these limits is termed the 'ischaemic penumbra'.[6] Tissue exposed to blood flow rates within this range is characterised by the potential for functional recovery without morphological damage, provided that local blood flow can be re-established at a sufficient level and within a certain time. The duration of impairment in blood flow that can be tolerated is also dependent on the severity of associated metabolic disturbances. As a consequence, the theory of a 'therapeutic window' has been postulated – a duration of time during which effective restoration of blood flow and intervention to prevent the consequences of biochemical alterations can be successful in ensuring the viability of cerebral tissue.

This review will discuss the basic mechanisms of ischaemia and the hypothesis of the therapeutic window. The relevance of experimental results concerning these parameters to the clinical management of stroke is highlighted.

1. Flow Thresholds for Functional and Morphological Integrity

As mentioned in the introduction to this review, two ischaemic flow thresholds exist – one defines functional damage and the other morphological damage.

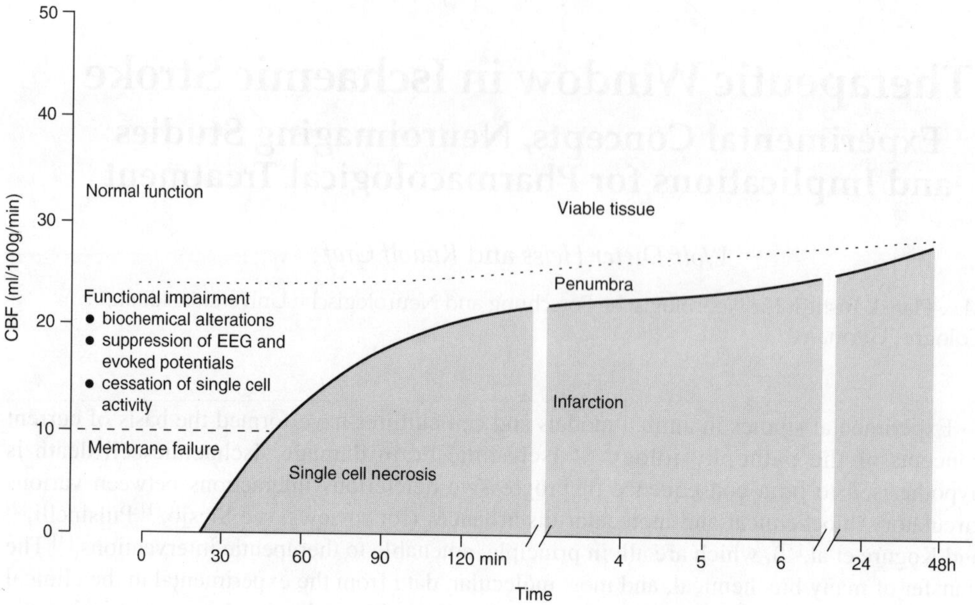

Fig. 1. Diagram of cerebral blood flow (CBF) thresholds required for the preservation of function and morphology of brain tissue. The development of single cell necrosis and infarction is dependent on the duration of time for which CBF is impaired below a certain level. The solid line separates structurally damaged from functionally impaired but morphologically intact tissue (the 'penumbra'), and the dashed line distinguishes viable from functionally impaired tissue.

1.1 Functional Damage

The functional threshold was demonstrated in monkeys exposed to ischaemia. A reduction in blood flow led to the gradual development of a neurological deficit, progressing from mild pareses at a flow rate of 22 ml/100g/min to complete paralysis at a rate of 8 ml/100g/min.[7] Concurrently, the electrocorticogram and evoked potentials were abolished at a flow rate of 15 to 20 ml/100g/min,[8,9] and the spontaneous activity of cortical neurons disappeared at approximately 18 ml/100g/min.[10] There was a large variability in the functional threshold of individual neurons, indicating selective vulnerability.[11]

Biochemical substrates and markers follow similar threshold dependencies. However, the pattern is more complex and the threshold values fall within a larger range, suggesting a specific role of individual metabolites in the development of ischaemic injury (for a review see Hossmann[12]). With declining flow rates (from the normal cortical values of 60 to 100 ml/100g/min, depending on species), protein synthesis is inhibited at about 55 ml/100g/min,[13] followed by a stimulation of anaerobic glycolysis at 35 ml/100g/min,[14] the release of neurotransmitters[15] and the disturbance of energy metabolism[16] at about 20 ml/100g/min, and finally the terminal depolarisation and concomitant potassium efflux at 15 ml/100g/min.[17]

1.2 Morphological Damage

Whereas neuronal function is impaired immediately blood flow drops below the threshold, the development of irreversible morphological damage is time dependent. Once morphological damage becomes apparent, the initially reversible functional deficit develops into a persistent defect. Numerous studies have investigated the duration for which brain tissue or individual cells can tolerate ischaemia of a given intensity (reviewed by Heiss[5]).

The interaction of severity and duration of ischaemia in the development of irreversible cell damage can be studied by simultaneous recordings of cortical neuronal activity and local blood flow.[11] On the basis of a large number of neurons assessed during and after ischaemia of varying degree and duration, it is possible, despite the high variability of ischaemic tolerance, to construct a discriminant curve representing the worst possible constellations of residual blood flow and duration of ischaemia that still permit neuronal recovery. Typical points on this curve are blood flow rates of approximately 0, 10 or 15 ml/100g/min maintained for periods of 25, 40 and 80 minutes, respectively. Between 17 and 18 ml/100g/min, the duration of tolerated ischaemia tends to infinity, indicating that this flow state can lead to morphological damage but only when maintained for very long, as yet undefined, periods of time. These conditions of dense or prolonged ischaemia predict cell damage that may take the form of large infarcts or single cell necroses.

Interspecies differences must be taken into consideration when experimental results are compared. In monkeys and cats, large infarcts develop with residual flow rates of 12 ml/100g/min lasting for 2 to 3 hours,[7,18,19] and individual cells may become necrotic at lower flow values after shorter periods of time.[20,21] However, middle cerebral artery (MCA) occlusion in rats induced selective neuronal necrosis in the caudate/putamen after only 15 minutes, localised infarcts in the caudate/putamen and selective neuronal necrosis in the neocortex after 30 minutes, and cortical infarcts after 60 minutes. With an occlusion time of 120 to 180 minutes, infarct size increased and reached that found after permanent MCA occlusion.[22]

Additionally, morphological tolerance to ischaemia is affected by various inherent or external factors: hypertensive rats are less tolerant than normotensive rats,[23] and tolerance is dependent on the number of ischaemic episodes[24] and body temperature.[25] It must also be kept in mind that delayed neuronal death after reperfusion may result from selective vulnerability of neurons.

2. The Ischaemic Penumbra

The term 'ischaemic penumbra' was originally applied to brain tissue perfused at values between the functional and morphological thresholds.[6] However, the term has recently been extended to characterise ischaemically affected but still viable tissue that has an uncertain likelihood for infarction or recovery.[26] The hypothesis of the ischaemic penumbra has been developed from animal experiments, and so its relationship to the clinical situation is not always clear.

Penumbra tissue has had blood flow decreased to the point of causing electrophysiological silence and transient, recurrent losses of membrane ion gradients and energy metabolites.[27] In such tissue, blood flow is decreased below the metabolic demand, but energy metabolism is preserved at a level allowing morphological preservation of tissue ('misery perfusion').[28]

However, continuing ischaemic stress and/or additional energy demanding episodes will exhaust this limited capacity and transform penumbra into necrotic tissue.

Results have accumulated supporting the concept of the ischaemic penumbra as a dynamic process of impaired perfusion and unstable energy metabolism, eventually propagating from the centre of ischaemia to the neighbouring tissue, with the potential of recovery, or progressive necrosis and growing infarction.

2.1 Mediators of Ischaemic Damage

The processes involved in the propagation of ischaemic damage are outlined in figure 2. Various markers, mediators and modulators of ischaemic penumbra have been suggested, including:

- waves of depolarisation
- increases in the extracellular levels of excitatory amino acids
- activation of calcium (Ca^{++}) channels
- induction of immediate early genes and expression of heat shock proteins.

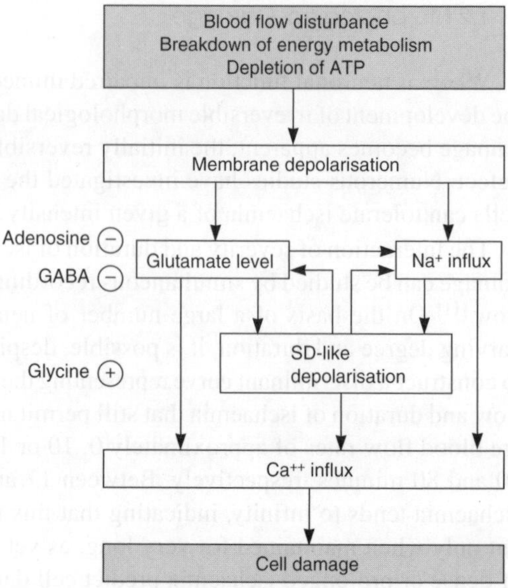

Fig. 2. Simplified diagram of the major factors involved in the development of ischaemic damage.
ATP = adenosine triphosphate; **GABA** = γ-aminobutyric acid; **SD** = spreading depression.

Some of these processes can be affected by therapeutic interventions.

In the ischaemic core, the tissue depolarises permanently within a few minutes. However, waves of transient neuronal depolarisation resembling spreading depression are regularly seen in peri-infarct tissue, especially in small animals like rats and gerbils. Nedergaard and Hansen[29] have differentiated between short lasting (spreading depressions) and longer lasting ischaemic depolarisations in focal ischaemia. The former are possibly evoked in the ischaemic core by extracellular potassium and/or glutamate; the latter may be elicited by multiple foci of reduced blood flow within the ischaemic border zones. In rats, a significant correlation was detected between infarct volume and number of depolarisations.[30]

Spreading depressions under nonischaemic conditions are paralleled by transient increases in the extracellular level of excitatory amino acids.[31] The blockade of *N*-methyl-D-aspartate (NMDA) receptors by dizocilpine (MK-801) reduces or abolishes waves of spreading depression in penumbral cortical regions and also reduces the volume of infarcts.[32,33] A corresponding effect on both the number of spreading depressions and volume of infarct was found with hypothermia.[34] It was therefore suggested[12] that the limited survival of the penumbra is due to peri-infarct depolarisations, which result in repeated episodes of tissue hypoxia. This is a result of the increased metabolic work load not being coupled to an adequate increase of collateral blood supply.[35]

The influx of Ca^{++} into cells is thought to play a key role in immediate as well as delayed cell damage.[36] The flow threshold for Ca^{++} accumulation is similar to that for electrical failure. During reperfusion, the time course of Ca^{++} accumulation is predictive of the fate of the tissue: further increases in Ca^{++} levels occur in areas found to be severely damaged on subsequent histological examination, whereas tissue remains histologically intact when Ca^{++} level normalises with reperfusion.[37]

The early excessive Ca^{++} influx associated with ischaemia could be caused by NMDA receptor–mediated Ca^{++} channel opening. This is evidenced by the finding that the resulting neuronal damage can be prevented by dizocilpine, but not by voltage-sensitive Ca^{++} channel antagonists such as nimodipine and nicardipine, despite the action of the latter drugs on cellular energy metabolism.[38,39]

[^{11}C]Nimodipine can be used as an indicator of ischaemically disturbed but viable, i.e. penumbra, tissue, because it clearly labels activated Ca^{++} channels.[40] Binding of [^{11}C]nimodipine is increased early after ischaemia, and later reduced, in penumbra tissue. These time-dependent cyclic changes of receptor channel activation and deactivation progress from the ischaemic centre to the periphery. The delay in the onset of this cycle and the final state of the tissue is related to the severity and duration of ischaemia in a respective region.

The release of excitatory amino acids and the activation of the respective receptors and receptor-operated ion channels during ischaemia is a key mechanism in the biochemical/molecular cascade leading to tissue damage. Most research in this respect has shifted from *in vitro* investigations on cultured nerve cells and brain slices to systemic animal experiments in which global and focal ischaemia has been induced,[41] and from the observation of particular and selectively vulnerable structures, i.e. the hippocampus, to studies of brain structures relevant for clinical stroke, i.e. cortex and basal ganglia.

Increases in the levels of excitatory and inhibitory amino acid neurotransmitters in the cortex also follow a typical flow threshold pattern.[42] This is not observed for nontransmitter amino acids. The magnitude of glutamate release during ischaemia was positively correlated with infarct volume.[43,44] During transient short ischaemic episodes, the extracellular glutamate levels reached are below a critical level,[45] and reuptake systems for excitatory neurotransmitter amino acids or inhibitory neurotransmitters such as γ-aminobutyric acid (GABA) and adenosine[46] may inhibit the deleterious excitotoxic action of excitatory transmitters. However, in prolonged ischaemia, excitotoxicity may be enhanced by a slowly increasing glycine level and the early reduction in the levels of adenosine.[47] It must be considered, however, that increases in the levels of excitatory neurotransmitters in the periphery of ischaemia may not necessarily be a result of the generation of neuroactive amino acids within this region. Instead, it could be a result of leakage from the ischaemic core.[48] This effect has been demonstrated in the white matter and the CSF.[49]

The above findings might justify the speculation that a dynamic penumbra contributes to the progressive development of infarction: in prolonged ischaemia, an elevation of the levels of excitotoxic substances is sustained and the compounds might diffuse into the brain areas that are oligemic during the early phase of ischaemia. If not sufficiently inhibited, the deleterious cycle of ischaemic damage, including activation of Ca^{++} channels, is triggered, leading to a further increase of excitotoxic compounds that can diffuse into neighbouring areas.

2.2 Potential Therapeutic Interventions

Interference with the effect of excitatory amino acids and blockade of the respective receptors and ion channels appears to be a promising rationale for limiting ischaemic injury to the brain. Several strategies have been adopted for this purpose.[50] For example, NMDA receptors have been targeted, and several drugs that are antagonists of these receptors or sites on these receptors are currently in clinical trials for stroke, such as aptiganel, dextrorphan, selfotel, eliprodil and gavestinel (GV 150526A).[51] In addition, the use of Ca^{++} antagonists as treatments for stroke has been investigated. Nimodipine is the agent for which the most data are available, although others such as nicardipine and flunarizine have also been studied.[51] However, the results with these agents are controversial and clinical data are scarce.

3. Clinical Evidence of an Ischaemic Penumbra

The assessment of pathophysiological changes leading to ischaemic cell damage in a clinical setting is extremely difficult, as most of the biochemical markers used in preclinical studies cannot be determined in patients. Furthermore, most techniques for clinical examination do not provide information about the viability of tissue, and routine techniques that do allow assessment of physiological variables [e.g. positron emission tomography (PET), single photon emission computed tomography (SPECT), x-ray computed tomography, magnetic resonance imaging (MRI) and magnetic resonance spectroscopy] are unsuitable because of their logistic complexity.

Magnetic resonance spectroscopy is still in the preclinical testing stage.[52] However, pertinent findings of pathophysiological changes occurring during the early period after ischaemic stroke have been obtained by multitracer PET. This provides quantitative 'maps' of several important physiological variables, including regional cerebral blood flow (rCBF), regional blood volume, regional cerebral metabolic rate of oxygen ($rCMRO_2$) and regional cerebral metabolic rate of glucose ($rCMR_{glc}$). These studies conclude that tissue with $rCMRO_2$ below 65 μmol/100g/min and/or rCBF below 12 ml/100g/min definitely becomes necrotic.[53,54] Regions with rCBF between 12 and 22 ml/100g/min have an unstable metabolic function, and are considered to be the penumbra zone, because infarction will occur in such a region if low flow values persist.[55] Patients with transitory ischaemic attacks have a minimum rCBF value of 22 ml/100g/min.[56]

Uncoupled changes of flow and metabolism indicate the existence of viable but insufficiently supplied tissue in an ischaemic region: early perfusion failure manifests as a decrease in rCBF, with $rCMRO_2$ and $rCMR_{glc}$ remaining relatively preserved. This condition, termed 'misery perfusion',[28] implies that blood flow is inadequate relative to the metabolic energy demand for oxygen and other substrates for viable tissue. The observations in early stroke suggest that tissue affected by misery perfusion, but with $rCMRO_2$ still above the critical threshold, is viable and may recover.[57,58] However, the few published studies showed that most penumbra zones that had increased oxygen extraction fraction (OEF) turned into infarction in the period after a stroke.

In a repeat multitracer PET study of patients who had had an acute ischaemic stroke,[59] differentiation between the ischaemic core and periphery demonstrated that viable but misery perfused tissue exists in the border zone of ischaemia up to 48 hours after stroke. Only in a few regions, or in special cases with increased OEF and slightly impaired $rCMRO_2$, was

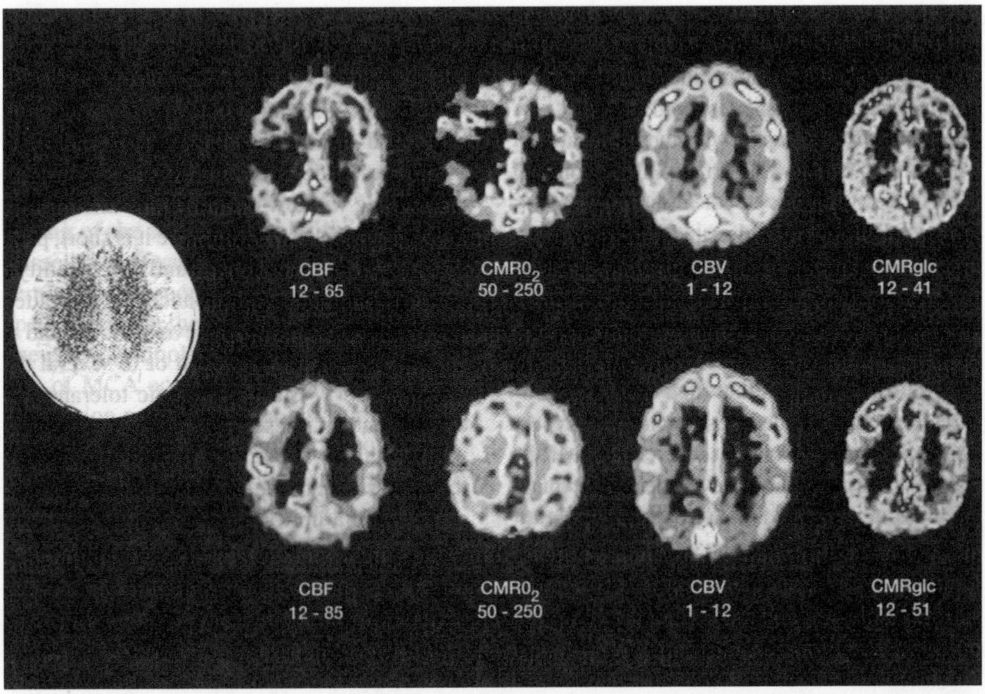

Fig. 3. Data from 2 positron emission tomography scans in a patient who recovered completely from hemiparalysis after an ischaemic stroke. The scans were taken 10 hours after the onset of hemiplegia (**top line**) and 10 days after the stroke (**bottom line**). A severe decrease in cerebral blood flow (CBF) in the first scan can be seen to have developed into hyperperfusion at the second scan. Regional cerebral metabolic rate of oxygen ($CMRO_2$) and regional cerebral metabolic rate of glucose (CMR_{glc}) remain above a critical level. A late scan (taken 10 days after the attack) showed that gross infarction had not developed. **CBV** = cerebral blood volume.

metabolism preserved close to normal values, and tissue remained morphologically intact (see fig. 3 for an example of such a case). Most tissue compartments showing misery perfusion in the first day, suffered progressive metabolic derangement and became necrotic during the following 2 weeks.

Whereas the viable peri-infarct penumbra tissue exhibits some potential for effective treatment, available therapeutic options, in most cases, cannot prevent subsequent progression to necrosis. Some studies, however, suggest that hyperperfusion occurring early after the ischaemic attack and affecting tissue that has undergone little metabolic alteration is associated with good recovery.[60-62] This result suggests the beneficial effect of early reperfusion, and is the basis for interventional thrombolytic therapy, by which outcome after basilar and MCA occlusion can be significantly improved.[63-66]

In rare cases of carotid stenosis, low perfusion is accompanied by increased OEF indicative of a state of chronic misery perfusion or penumbra.[67,68] Such single cases described occasionally in the past may form a rationale for bypass surgery, by which flow and metabolism can be effectively increased.[69,70] However, the clinical impact of such a treatment remains controversial.[71]

4. Techniques for Assessing Ischaemic Damage

4.1 Positron Emission Tomography: Correlation Between Animal Models and the Clinical Situation

In the clinical setting, only a few of the many factors contributing to the complex process of ischaemic tissue damage, such as blood flow, blood volume, oxygen consumption and glucose metabolism, can be assessed by functional imaging techniques. Additionally, clinical studies are restricted to anecdotal time points in the course of the disease. The complicated logistics involved in the regional determination of physiological variables prevent their repeated evaluation early after an ischaemic attack, which is when the fate of the patient is decided. Therefore, a gap exists between the results obtained at well defined but usually singular time points in animal experiments on the one hand, and the findings collected incidentally in patients at various times after the onset of stroke on the other. Animal experiments are necessary to better understand the results of multitracer PET studies involving patients early after a stroke. In these experiments, regional changes in physiological variables can be followed, from the vascular attack to the permanent defective state, and then related to histological alterations.

With advanced PET equipment, it has become feasible to study pathophysiological changes in brain perfusion and metabolism after MCA occlusion in animals, such as baboons[72,73] and cats.[74,75] Tenjin et al.[72] observed a severe reduction of CBF (to below 18 ml/100g/min) and a significant increase of OEF 1 hour after occlusion in the core of ischaemia, and a decrease of OEF 9 hours after occlusion. However, Pappata et al.[73] reported that the decrease of CBF in the territory of the occluded vessel in baboons was not so severe (21% at 1 hour and 31% at 3 to 4 hours after occlusion).

In these experiments, $CMRO_2$ was variable and declined 3 to 4 hours after MCA occlusion, but was only moderately reduced in regions with maximal OEF, suggesting prolonged viability. When the animals were followed after MCA occlusion,[76] infarcts were observed in the deep MCA territory, but not in the cortical regions. Changes of $CMRO_2$ occurred earlier and were more severe in the deep MCA territory than in the cortical regions. The infarcts in this model increased in size over several days.[77]

In cats, CBF, $CMRO_2$, OEF and CMR_{glc} were followed from control values before ischaemia to the endpoint of infarction 24 hours after MCA occlusion.[74] CBF within the MCA territory fell immediately upon arterial occlusion to below 30% of control, whereas $CMRO_2$ was less diminished and consequently OEF was increased, thus indicating misery perfusion. This ischaemic penumbra spread with time from the centre to the borders of the MCA territory. In most instances, the misery perfusion condition was followed by a marked decrease in OEF, reflecting progressive impairment of blood flow and metabolism and suggesting transition to necrosis. The infarcts were more or less complete 18 to 24 hours after MCA occlusion. Occasionally, spontaneous collateral reperfusion resolved the penumbra condition and morphological integrity of the cortex was preserved.

Reversible MCA occlusion was studied in cats,[78] with reopening of the MCA after 30, 60 or 120 minutes. All cats survived 30 minutes of MCA occlusion. OEF remained elevated throughout the ischaemic episode in the animals surviving 24 hours of reperfusion. However, the initial OEF increase disappeared during 60 minutes of ischaemia in those cats that died during the reperfusion period (fig. 4). In the cats that died during the observation period,

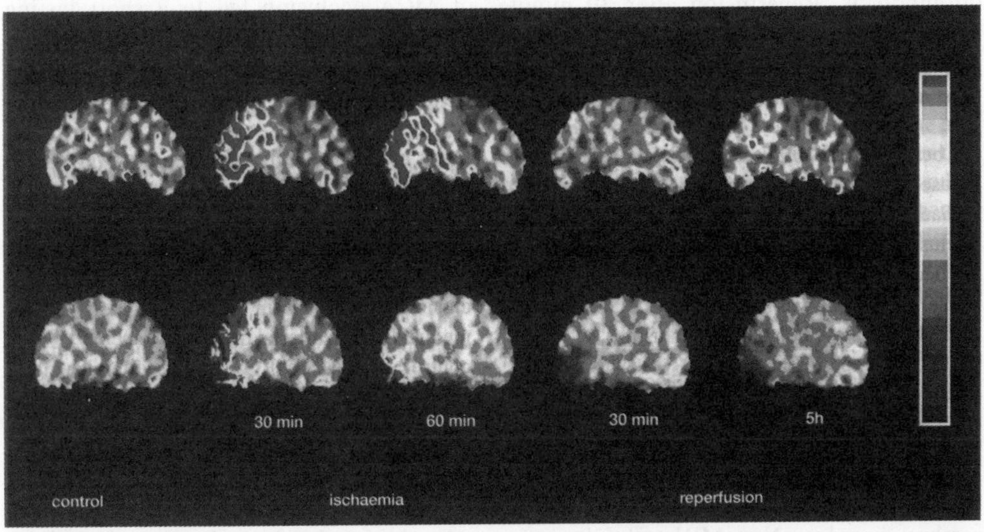

Fig. 4. Variable development of oxygen extraction fraction (OEF) during ischemia and reperfusion in 2 cats during the 24-hour observation period after middle cerebral artery occlusion and reperfusion. One cat survived (**top line**) while the other died (**bottom line**). Note the dynamic deterioration of OEF in the cat that died, as compared with an almost complete recovery in the surviving cat.

extended post-ischaemic hyperperfusion accompanied large defects of $CMRO_2$ and CMR_{glc}, large infarcts developed, and intracranial pressure increased fatally.[79] In the baboon MCA occlusion model, where ischaemia is less severe, longer periods of ischaemia were tolerated, and reopening of the vessels after 6 hours improved outcome and significantly reduced the size of the final infarcts.[80] These results further highlight the importance of the severity of ischaemia in relation to its duration for the further course after reperfusion.[10,11]

These PET studies demonstrate that the penumbra is a dynamic process. The time window for the eventual recovery of tissue – important as the therapeutic window – is therefore different for the core of dense ischaemia (where it is short, probably below 1 hour in the cat) and the vicinity with graded perfusional disturbance. In the latter, the time window is certainly several hours and might extend to 24 hours in the cat or to several days in the monkey.[77] Since ischaemic tolerance is species dependent, these data are relevant to the findings in human stroke where misery perfused, potentially viable tissue was found in the border zone of ischaemia up to 18[57,60] or even 48[59] hours after the attack, and misery perfused territories (fig. 3) were reperfused without a resultant infarction and functional deficit.[57,58]

PET studies in animal models simulate the course of perfusional and metabolic disturbances characteristic of ischaemic stroke in humans, and so a comparison of experimental results to clinical findings may be justified. Permanent MCA occlusion resembles the natural course after vascular occlusion, leading to large infarcts in most cases, with a chance of collateral reperfusion that may resolve misery perfusion and improve outcome. Reopening of the MCA resembles the (spontaneous) dissolution of vascular occlusions in transient ischaemic attacks, spontaneous lysis of emboli after a period beyond the tolerable time period, and therapeutic thrombolysis. Reperfusion after 30 minutes of MCA occlusion led to a short lasting hyperperfusion period and to a fast normalisation of flow and metabolism. This may be comparable with a transient ischaemic attack. During MCA occlusion of longer duration two patterns can be distinguished: (i) a decrease of the OEF during the time of MCA occlusion reflects fast irreversible damage of tissue, whereas (ii) the persistence of raised OEF indicates preserved viability of tissue over the ischaemic period. Forced reperfusion by reopening of the MCA cannot salvage already irreversibly damaged tissue, but may cause additional damage by inducing oedema via leaking vascular endothelium. In such cases, the infarcts are large and animals die early due to increased intracranial pressure. These courses resemble the deleterious outcome of thrombolytic therapy that is initiated too late and so could not prevent the development of large infarcts, resulting in additional oedema and secondary haemorrhagic transformation.

4.2 Magnetic Resonance Imaging:Use in Early Stroke

Of the available imaging techniques, MRI has the highest spatial resolution for detecting lesions in the brain, and has therefore gained a prominent position in the diagnosis of focal cerebral disorders. New MRI technologies provide additional information on pathophysiological and functional alterations, making this method a versatile tool with multiple applications.

In the management of acute stroke, a technique is needed which is readily available in the acute clinical setting, rapid, non-invasive and provides results rapidly. The latter is important to ensure that the necessary multiple diagnostic measurements are available within minutes, so as not to delay treatment beyond the optimal time window.[81]

Diffusion-weighted imaging (DWI) has considerable potential, as substantial changes in the parenchymal diffusion of water after the onset of ischaemia can be detected by this method. Since the detection of ischaemic stroke by DWI-MRI within minutes after experimental vascular occlusion was first demonstrated,[82] this technique has evolved as an important tool for both the identification of very early injury in patients and the quantitative assessment of the severity and volume of ischaemically compromised tissue.[83] In ischaemia models involving small animals (e.g. rats, gerbils, cats), DWI has been shown to be useful as an early diagnostic marker of ischaemia. It can also provide quantitative data on a physiological parameter [the apparent diffusion coefficient (ADC) of water in tissue] and volumetric analysis of the lesion. ADC values derived from DWI measurements can give a value for assessing the severity of ischaemic changes and also for following the time course in the evolution of irreversible damage.

DWI shows the area of reduced diffusion as a hyperintense region, which follows the redistribution of water from the extracellular to intracellular space as a consequence of reduced adenosine triphosphate (ATP)ase activity.[84] In the core of this area, ATP remains depleted, indicating necrotic transformation due to severely reduced perfusion.[85] Since disturbances of the water/ionic homeostasis occur immediately with disruptions of perfusion, DWI is able to detect the initial disturbance in ischaemia, and also shows the reversal of these alterations with early recovery. With this technique, the progression of ischaemic injury from areas of dense to those of moderate to mild flow decreases can be followed. In one study, the changes in DWI signals correlated with histological defects and metabolic abnormalities as assessed by autoradiographic and chemical imaging procedures at follow-up.[86]

ADC values change over the course of ischaemia, and there is also a gradual decrease in values from the periphery to the core of an ischaemic territory.[87] The threshold for ATP depletion, calculated by matching ADC to rCBF, was around 18 ml/100g/min. This is equal to 77% of control ADC and corresponded to previously described values. Tissue acidosis was observed in neighbouring, less affected areas.[85]

Reperfusion after transient MCA occlusion resulted in reversible signal changes in DWI; infarction only developed if the signal intensity ratio between ischaemic and non-ischaemic tissue rose above 1.46 during occlusion, even when it subsequently returned to near control.[88] It was also shown that the hyperintensity in DWI is less marked after 1 hour than after 2 hours of MCA occlusion,[89] and that hyperintensity observed during the reperfusion period can predict the size of the final infarct. When ADC progressively decreased despite reperfusion, a large infarction developed,[90] whereas ADC above a certain value predicted recovery. In addition, a relationship was found between quantitative change of diffusion – indicative of risk of injury – and the length of this disturbance, both of which predicted demarcated tissue injury.[91] These results indicate that DWI can be utilised to detect penumbra tissue.

With DWI techniques, the relationship between the number of spreading depression–like depolarisations (detected as transient decreases in ADC),[92] and infarct size[30] could be confirmed. The ADC-defined ischaemic region increased during 15 minute epochs by 37% with single spreading depressions and by 40% with multiple spreading depressions, whereas without spreading depressions an increase of only 14% was seen.[93] As a consequence, the final infarcts caused by MCA occlusion in rats were significantly larger when spreading depressions occurred.

Some of the compromised tissue can be salvaged by neuroprotective drugs and the effect – a decrease of the DWI lesion size after drug application, or continued growth in the untreated group – can be predicted in sequential MR images.[94,95] Antagonists of the NMDA receptor prevent spontaneously occurring and chemically elicited spreading depressions, and thereby mitigate the extent of ATP depletion (26 versus 49% of hemisphere),[96] decrease infarct size (49 versus 66% of hemisphere;[96] 54 versus 217mm^3[97]) and improve post-ischaemic perfusion and clinical outcome.[97]

The relevance of these results and the application of this elegant technology to the clinical setting, however, is still limited by technical and procedural problems. The echoplanear MRI equipment necessary for fast DWI and perfusion-weighted imaging is not available in all institutions that are involved in the treatment of acute stroke, and the procedure is difficult to execute in severely ill patients. Additionally, the accurate quantitation of ADC that is necessary for defining cellular viability and detecting salvageable ischaemic tissue is difficult to achieve,[98,99] and requires complex procedures including T_2-weighted images.[100]

Despite these procedural complexities which continue to limit broad clinical applications of the technique, the initial experience gathered in a few centres is promising.[101] Recent applications of DWI in patients early after ischaemic stroke indicated that decreased ADC is a marker of energy failure and identifies the penumbra.[102-104] Hyperintensive regions of decreased ADC identified ischaemic lesions that subsequently developed infarction less than 6 hours after onset.[105] The time course of these changes – initially 56% of control ADC, slowly increasing and reaching normal values within 5 to 10 days – also permitted the discrimination of acute lesions adjacent to chronic infarcts.[105,106] Together with T_2-weighted images, this yielded signatures that identified tissue that recovered, tissue in progression to necrosis and tissue already irreversibly damaged.[107]

Combined diffusion- and perfusion-weighted MRI can detect tissue that is at the greatest risk for the development of infarction, and might guide therapeutic interventions. Infarcts evolve over time into areas defined as the penumbra on earlier scans, and partial resolution of DWI abnormalities were observed after stroke without the development of infarction, both spontaneously or, in single cases, following administration of an NMDA receptor antagonist.[83] Even the final volume of infarction can be predicted, and the effect of a drug in reducing this lesion volume can be demonstrated.[108]

DW-MRI could become the most rapid and widely applied method of identifying tissue at high risk of infarction (the penumbra) and determining, on an individual basis, how long after the onset of stroke, therapies can be applied and still be effective. With the rapid advances in MRI technologies, it can be expected that these methods will be introduced into routine clinical practice in the near future. They will ensure that staging and predicting the progression of ischaemic damage become prerequisites for the treatment of stroke.

Compared with the high potential of DW-MRI, the role of magnetic resonance spectroscopy, which is of significant scientific value, is still limited in the clinical management of acute ischaemic stroke.[52]

5. Application of Therapeutic Windows to the Treatment of Ischaemic Stroke

Experimental data suggest that the extent of neurological deficits is dependent on the severity and duration of flow impairment, and that complex biochemical and molecular mechanisms are involved in the development and progression of ischaemic damage. These data point to several time windows during which therapeutic strategies must be initiated.

From animal experiments and preliminary clinical data, it may be deducted that a short therapeutic window of a few hours after the onset of ischaemia is relevant for the re-establishment of perfusion. However, the time-dependent propagation of the ischaemic penumbra suggests an extended period during which there may be effective intervention with agents that interrupt the biochemical/molecular processes associated with ischaemia. In clinical reality, both rationales must be utilised for the effective treatment of stroke, and it is likely that various strategies will be combined in the future.

It should be noted that animal studies have provided information on the existence and duration of a therapeutic window. If these findings are ignored and clinical stroke trials are performed with patient entry beyond the therapeutic window, the efficacy of a treatment regimen cannot be verified. Therefore, criteria tested in animal models should be considered when clinical trials are designed.[109]

5.1 Therapeutic Window for the Re-Establishment of Perfusion

In clinical studies that have evaluated the influence of time to spontaneous reperfusion,[110] recanalisation within 8 hours in conjunction with good transcortical collateralisation was found to have a favourable impact on infarct size and clinical outcome. In contrast, recanalisation times greater than 8 hours always caused lesions that extended to the cortex. When initiated 4 to 6 hours after the onset of stroke symptoms, thrombolytic therapy recanalised 21 to 59%

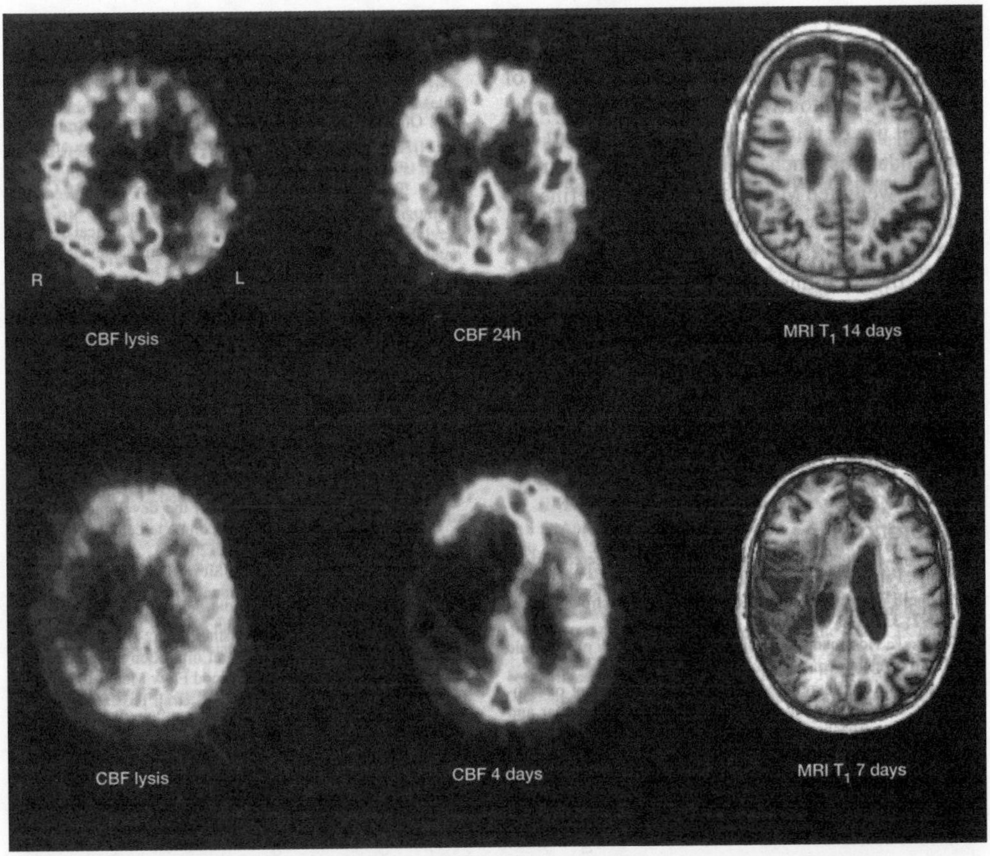

Fig. 5. Examples of positron emission cerebral blood flow (CBF) and magnetic resonance imaging (MRI) scans in 2 patients undergoing thrombolytic therapy after ischaemic stroke. **Top line:** successful reperfusion and full clinical recovery without infarction in a 70-year-old male patient who presented with a complete right sensomotoric hemisyndrome and global aphasia. **Bottom line:** failure of recanalisation and poor outcome with severe neurological defect and large infarction in a 76-year-old male who presented with severe left sensorimotor syndrome. Note the difference of spontaneous collateral perfusion before lysis.

of occluded vessels in the carotid territory and 40 to 55% of occluded basilar arteries.[111] Two small placebo-controlled studies of carotid territory stroke indicated a clinical benefit from fibrinolysis,[63,64] and this result was supported in two large multicentre trials.[65,66] After successful lysis of an occluded basilar artery, patients had a 50% chance of survival (compared with 10% without recanalisation), with minor to moderate associated neurological deficits.[112] The therapeutic window relevant for the re-establishment of sufficient flow and accessible to thrombolysis and other perfusion-based therapies is only a few hours, with a limit usually set at 3 hours. Indeed, the US Food and Drug Administration has recently approved the use of alteplase as a treatment for acute stroke, but only when administered within 3 hours of symptom onset.

Despite the proven successes of thrombolysis, not all patients who achieve effective reperfusion are improved, with a varying percentage experiencing poor outcome after the development of space-occupying infarction[113] and secondary haemorrhage.[114,115] In this context, the efficacy of thrombolytic therapy is related to the existence of 'penumbral' tissue perfused at rates below the functional threshold, yet above the level indicating or leading to irreversible morphological damage.

In order to further analyse the influence of residual perfusion on outcome, regional cerebral perfusion was studied at the start (<3 hours after onset of symptoms) and repeatedly after thrombolytic therapy (alteplase 0.9 mg/kg according to a National Institute of Neurological Diseases and Stroke protocol)[66] in patients with an acute hemispheric stroke.[116] After 3-dimensional alignment and normalisation on the mean of the contralateral hemisphere, the relative perfusion rates of first and second measurements were related to defects found in late T_1-weighted MRI on a voxel-by-voxel basis. Before initiation of thrombolytic therapy, all patients showed marked hypoperfusion of their affected MCA territory (fig. 5). Within these hypoperfused areas, volumes of tissue at risk of ischaemic damage were operationally defined as <50% uptake of the contralateral mean, representing tissue below or above the viability threshold, respectively. Patients in whom large proportions of ischaemically compromised tissue were effectively reperfused, and not included in the final infarct identified on late MRI, recovered completely or experienced slight damage; those in whom recanalisation reached less than half the deficiently supplied territory had an unfavourable outcome with severe permanent defects. These findings indicate that residual flow in the given time interval is the crucial prognostic factor for thrombolytic therapy. However, it has to be further analysed whether higher residual blood flow values would justify an extended time window for thrombolysis.

5.2 Therapeutic Window for the Inhibition of Biochemical/Molecular Changes

The existence of a window of longer duration, during which agents could be given that interfere with the biochemical and molecular disturbances associated with ischaemia, is still controversial.[117-120] Furthermore, the duration of the window cannot be easily deducted from a beneficial effect of therapeutic strategies. Further controlled studies need to be carried out to prove convincingly the value of therapies such as those that:[121]

- interfere with increased Ca^{++} entry into cells
- inhibit amino acid excitotoxicity
- scavenge free-radicals
- affect nitric oxide synthetase.

There are a few examples indicating that interaction with such mechanisms may result in an improved outcome after a cerebrovascular attack. Furthermore, it appears that PET is able to identify early pathophysiological changes that occur after ischaemic stroke, and predict treatment effects and outcome. Therefore, PET and DW-MRI might be of value for the demonstration of viable tissue and of treatment effects in patients with stroke.

Ca^{++} antagonists were able to improve neurological outcome and reduce histological damage in animal experiments and therefore have been used in ischaemic stroke. The results of multicentre trials have been controversial and benefits were only indicated in a meta-analysis;[122] beneficial outcome was obtained only when treatment was started within the first 12 hours after the onset of symptoms. In multitracer PET studies,[55] nimodipine was found to be effective in reversing the decline in $CMRO_2$ and increasing CBF in the densely ischaemic zone, whereas in the penumbra $CMRO_2$ was improved, but the difference compared with the control group was not statistically significant. In another study,[123] PET demonstrated that $rCMR_{glc}$ in the cortex of the hemisphere outside the infarct improved significantly within the first 3 weeks after the stroke in patients treated with nimodipine. Furthermore, patients in the treatment group reached higher scores in the Barthel-Index after 6 months.

These data may help to explain the controversial conclusions from the multicentre trials of nimodipine. The drug can only be effective as long as viable tissue is present in a progressive ischaemic lesion; when given after that period (which might be 12 hours), a therapeutic effect is unlikely to be achieved.

Similar results were obtained in a double-blind, controlled clinical trial with propentofylline, an adenosine reuptake inhibitor that counteracts glutamate excitotoxicity.[124] PET showed that $rCMR_{glc}$ increased significantly in the infarct and in the ipsilateral grey matter in the treatment groups compared with the placebo group. Perhaps of more therapeutic relevance was the significant difference in changes occurring in peri-infarct regions with increased OEF: at follow-up after 2 weeks, CBF, $CMRO_2$ and $rCMR_{glc}$ were less impaired in the treated than in the placebo patients. After 3 months these effects were reflected as differences in clinical recovery (change in Barthel-Index: propentofylline 45 points *vs* placebo 25 points). However, owing to the small number of patients in each group, these differences were not statistically significant ($p = 0.07$).

6. Conclusion

The existence of a therapeutic window for the restoration of blood flow after acute ischaemic stroke is evident from experimental studies and clinical experience. This has formed the basis for the early thrombolytic treatment (within 3 hours of the onset of symptoms) of stroke and thus for the successful use of this therapy. State-of-the-art imaging modalities, such as PET and diffusion- and perfusion-weighted MRI, have helped to define the therapeutic window in animal models of focal ischaemia and in patients who have experienced a stroke, by demonstrating the presence of ischaemically compromised but viable tissue. These techniques are also used to evaluate the success of thrombolytics and other therapeutic strategies that aim to achieve early interruption of the devastating molecular and biological alterations that are triggered during the ischaemic period.

References

1. Siesjö BK. Pathophysiology and treatment of focal cerebral ischemia. Part 1: Pathophysiology. J Neurosurg 1992; 77: 169-84
2. Pulsinelli W. Pathophysiology of acute ischaemic stroke. Lancet 1992; 339: 533-6
3. Kogure K, Hossmann K-A, Siesjö BK. Neurology of ischemic brain damage. Amsterdam: Elsevier, 1993
4. Ginsberg MD. Emerging strategies for the treatment of ischemic brain injury. In: Waxman SG, editor. Molecular and cellular approaches to the treatment of ischemic brain disease. New York: Raven Press, 1993: 207-37
5. Heiss WD. Experimental evidence for ischemic thresholds and functional recovery. Stroke 1992; 23: 1668-72
6. Astrup J, Siesjö BK, Symon L. Thresholds in cerebral ischemia – the ischemic penumbra. Stroke 1981; 12: 723-5
7. Jones TH, Morawetz RB, Crowell RM, et al. Thresholds of focal cerebral ischemia in awake monkeys. J Neurosurg 1981; 54: 773-82
8. Sharbrough FW, Messick JM, Sundt Jr TM. Correlation of continuous electroencephalograms with cerebral blood flow measurements during carotid endarterectomy. Stroke 1973; 4: 674-83
9. Branston NM, Symon L, Crockard HA, et al. Relationship between the cortical evoked potential and local cortical blood flow following acute middle cerebral artery occlusion in the baboon. Exp Neurol 1974; 45: 195-208
10. Heiss WD, Hayakawa T, Waltz AG. Cortical neuronal function during ischemia. Arch Neurol 1976; 33: 813-20
11. Heiss WD, Rosner G. Functional recovery of cortical neurons as related to degree and duration of ischemia. Ann Neurol 1983; 14: 294-301
12. Hossmann KA. Viability thresholds and the penumbra of focal ischemia. Ann Neurol 1994; 36: 557-65

13. Mies G, Ishimaru S, Xie Y, et al. Ischemic thresholds of cerebral protein synthesis and energy state following middle cerebral artery occlusion in rat. J Cereb Blood Flow Metab 1991; 11: 753-61
14. Paschen W, Mies G, Hossmann KA. Threshold relationship between cerebral blood flow, glucose utilization, and energy metabolites during development of stroke in gerbils. Exp Neurol 1992; 117: 325-33
15. Shimada N, Graf R, Rosner G, et al. Ischemic flow threshold for extracellular glutamate increase in cat cortex. J Cereb Blood Flow Metab 1989; 9: 603-6
16. Obrenovitch TP, Garofalo O, Harris RJ, et al. Brain tissue concentrations of ATP, phosphocreatine, lactate, and tissue pH in relation to reduced cerebral blood flow following experimental acute middle cerebral artery occlusion. J Cereb Blood Flow Metab 1988; 8: 866-74
17. Astrup J, Symon L, Branston NM, et al. Cortical evoked potential and extracellular K^+ and H^+ at critical levels of brain ischemia. Stroke 1977; 8: 51-7
18. Tamura A, Asano T, Sano K. Correlation between rCBF and histological changes following temporary middle cerebral artery occlusion. Stroke 1980; 11: 487-93
19. Marcoux FW, Morawetz RB, Crowell RM, et al. Differential regional vulnerability in transient focal cerebral ischemia. Stroke 1982; 13: 339-46
20. Pulsinelli WA, Brierley JB, Plum F. Temporal profile of neuronal damage in a model of transient forebrain ischemia. Ann Neurol 1982; 11: 491-8
21. Jenkins LW, Povlishock JT, Lewelt W, et al. The role of postischemic recirculation in the development of ischemic neuronal injury following complete cerebral ischemia. Acta Neuropathol 1981; 55: 205-20
22. Memezawa H, Smith ML, Siesjö BK. Penumbral tissues salvaged by reperfusion following middle cerebral artery occlusion in rats. Stroke 1992; 23: 552-9
23. Jacewicz M, Tanabe J, Pulsinelli WA. The CBF threshold and dynamics for focal cerebral infarction in spontaneously hypertensive rats. J Cereb Blood Flow Metab 1992; 12: 359-70
24. Tomida S, Nowak TS, Vass K, et al. Experimental model for repetitive ischemic attacks in the gerbil: the cumulative effect of repeated ischemic insults. J Cereb Blood Flow Metab 1987; 7: 773-82
25. Morikawa E, Ginsberg MD, Dietrich WD, et al. The significance of brain temperature in focal cerebral ischemia: histopathological consequences of middle cerebral artery occlusion in the rat. J Cereb Blood Flow Metab 1992; 12: 380-9
26. Heiss WD, Graf R. The ischemic penumbra. Curr Opin Neurol 1994; 7: 11-9
27. Ginsberg MD, Pulsinelli WA. The ischemic penumbra, injury thresholds, and the therapeutic window for acute stroke. Ann Neurol 1994; 36: 553-4
28. Baron JC, Bousser MG, Rey A, et al. Reversal of focal 'misery-perfusion syndrome' by extra-intracranial arterial bypass in hemodynamic cerebral ischemia. Stroke 1981; 12: 454-9
29. Nedergaard M, Hansen AJ. Characterization of cortical depolarizations evoked in focal cerebral ischemia. J Cereb Blood Flow Metab 1993; 13: 568-74
30. Mies G, Iijima T, Hossmann KA. Correlation between peri-infarct DC shifts and ischaemic neuronal damage in rat. Neuroreport 1993; 4: 709-11
31. Fabricius M, Jensen LH, Lauritzen M. Microdialysis of interstitial amino acids during spreading depression and anoxic depolarization in rat neocortex. Brain Res 1993; 612: 61-9
32. Gill R, Andine P, Hillered L, et al. The effect of MK-801 on cortical spreading depression in the penumbral zone following focal ischemia in the rat. J Cereb Blood Flow Metab 1992; 12: 371-9
33. Iijima T, Mies G, Hossmann KA. Repeated negative DC deflections in rat cortex following middle cerebral artery occlusion are abolished by MK-801: effect on volume of ischemic injury. J Cereb Blood Flow Metab 1992; 12: 727-33
34. Chen Q, Chopp M, Bodzin G, et al. Temperature modulation of cerebral depolarization during focal cerebral ischemia in rats: correlation with ischemic injury. J Cereb Blood Flow Metab 1993; 13: 389-94
35. Back T, Höhn-Berlage M, Kohno K, et al. Diffusion NMR imaging in experimental stroke: correlation with cerebral metabolites. Stroke 1994; 25: 494-500
36. Siesjö BK, Bengtsson F. Calcium fluxes, calcium antagonists, and calcium-related pathology in brain ischemia, hypoglycemia, and spreading depression. J Cereb Blood Flow Metab 1989; 9: 127-40
37. Uematsu D, Araki N, Greenberg JH, et al. Combined therapy with MK-801 and nimodipine for protection of ischemic brain damage. Neurology 1991; 41: 88-94
38. Nakamura K, Hatakeyama T, Furuta S, et al. The role of early Ca^{++} influx in the pathogenesis of delayed neuronal death after brief forebrain ischemia in gerbils. Brain Res 1993; 613: 181-92
39. Lemons BV, Chehrazi BB, Kauten R, et al. The effect of nimodipine on high-energy phosphates and intracellular pH during cerebral ischemia. J Neurotrauma 1993; 10: 73-81
40. Hakim AM, Hogan MJ. *In vivo* binding of nimodipine in the brain: I. The effect of focal cerebral ischemia. J Cereb Blood Flow Metab 1991; 11: 762-70
41. Choi DW. NMDA receptor, AMPA receptors, and extracellular acidity in ischemic brain damage: a view from the dish. In: Krieglstein J, Oberpichler-Schwenk H, editors. Pharmacology of cerebral ischemia. Stuttgart: Wiss Verl Ges, 1992: 45-52
42. Shimada N, Graf R, Rosner G, et al. Differences in ischemia-induced accumulation of amino acids in the cat cortex. Stroke 1990; 21: 1445-51

43. Takagi K, Ginsberg MD, Globus MY-T, et al. Changes in amino acid neurotransmitters and cerebral blood flow in the ischemic penumbral region following middle cerebral artery occlusion in the rat: correlation with histopathology. J Cereb Blood Flow Metab 1993; 13: 575-85
44. Taguchi J, Graf R, Rosner G, et al. Prolonged transient ischemia results in impaired CBF recovery and secondary glutamate accumulation in cats. J Cereb Blood Flow Metab 1996; 16: 271-9
45. Ueda Y, Obrenovitch TP, Lok SY, et al. Efflux of glutamate produced by short ischemia of varied severity in rat striatum. Stroke 1992; 23: 253-9
46. Matsumoto K, Graf R, Rosner G, et al. Flow thresholds for extracellular purine catabolite elevation in cat focal ischemia. Brain Res 1992; 579: 309-14
47. Matsumoto K, Graf R, Rosner G, et al. Elevation of neuroactive substances in the cortex of cats during prolonged focal ischemia. J Cereb Blood Flow Metab 1993; 13: 586-94
48. Obrenovitch TP, Urenjak J, Richards DA, et al. Extracellular neuroactive amino acids in the rat striatum during ischemia: comparison between penumbral conditions and ischaemia with sustained anoxic depolarisation. J Neurochem 1993; 61: 178-86
49. Shimada N, Graf R, Rosner G, et al. Ischemia-induced accumulation of extracellular amino acids in cerebral cortex, white matter, and cerebrospinal fluid. J Neurochem 1993; 60: 66-71
50. Pulsinelli W, Sarokin A, Buchan A. Antagonism of the NMDA and non-NMDA receptors in global versus focal brain ischemia. In: Kogure K, Hossmann KA, Siesjö BK, editors. Progress in brain research. Vol. 96. Amsterdam: Elsevier Science Publishers, 1993: 125-35
51. Dorman PJ, Counsell CE, Sandercock PAG. Recently developed neuroprotective therapies for acute stroke: a quantitative systemic review of clinical trials. CNS Drugs 1996; 5 (6): 457-74
52. Prichard JW. The role of magnetic resonance spectroscopy in stroke. In: Moskowitz MA, Caplan LR, editors. Cerebrovascular diseases. Boston: Butterworth-Heinemann, 1995: 475-85
53. Baron JC. Positron tomography in cerebral ischemia. Neuroradiology 1985; 27: 509-16
54. Powers WJ, Grubb Jr RL, Darriet D, et al. Cerebral blood flow and cerebral metabolic rate of oxygen requirements for cerebral function and viability in humans. J Cereb Blood Flow Metab 1985; 5: 600-8
55. Hakim AM, Evans AC, Berger L, et al. The effect of nimodipine on the evolution of human cerebral infarction studied by PET. J Cereb Blood Flow Metab 1989; 9: 523-34
56. Powers WJ, Press GW, Grubb Jr RL, et al. The effect of hemodynamically significant carotid artery disease on the hemodynamic status of the cerebral circulation. Ann Intern Med 1987; 106: 27-35
57. Furlan M, Marchal G, Viader F, et al. Spontaneous neurological recovery after stroke and the fate of the ischemic penumbra. Ann Neurol 1996; 40: 216-26
58. Heiss W-D, Fink GR, Huber M, et al. Positron emission tomography imaging and the therapeutic window. Stroke 1993; 24 Suppl. I: I50–3
59. Heiss W-D, Huber M, Fink G, et al. Progressive derangement of periinfarct viable tissue in ischemic stroke. J Cereb Blood Flow Metab 1992; 12: 193-203
60. Marchal G, Serrati C, Rioux P, et al. PET imaging of cerebral perfusion and oxygen consumption in acute ischaemic stroke: relation to outcome. Lancet 1993; 341: 925-7
61. Fink GR, Herholz K, Pietrzyk U, et al. Peri-infarct perfusion in human ischemia: its relation to tissue metabolism, morphology, and clinical outcome. J Stroke Cerebrovasc Dis 1993; 3: 123-31
62. Marchal G, Furlan M, Beaudouin V, et al. Early spontaneous hyperperfusion after stroke – a marker of favourable tissue outcome? Brain 1996; 119: 409-19
63. Mori E, Yoneda Y, Tabuchi M. Intravenous recombinant tissue plasminogen activator in acute carotid artery territory stroke. Neurology 1992; 42: 976-82
64. Yamaguchi T, Hayakawa T, Kiuchi H. Intravenous tissue plasminogen activator ameliorates the outcome of hyperacute embolic stroke. Cerebrovasc Dis 1993; 3: 269-72
65. Hacke W, Kaste M, Fieschi C, et al. Intravenous thrombolysis with recombinant tissue plasminogen activator for acute hemispheric stroke. The European Cooperative ECASS Study Group. JAMA 1995; 274: 1017-25
66. The National Institute of Neurological Disorders and Stroke rt-PA Stroke Study Group. Tissue plasminogen activator for acute ischemic stroke. N Engl J Med 1995; 333: 1581-7
67. Yamauchi H, Fukuyama H, Fujimoto N, et al. Significance of low perfusion with increased oxygen extraction fraction in a case of internal carotid artery stenosis. Stroke 1992; 23: 431-2
68. Yamauchi H, Fukuyama H, Nagahama Y, et al. Evidence of misery perfusion and risk for recurrent stroke in major cerebral arterial occlusive diseases from PET. J Neurol Neurosurg Psychiatry 1996; 61: 18-25
69. Ishikawa T, Yasui N, Suzuki A, et al. STA-MCA bypass surgery for internal carotid artery occlusion – comparative follow-up study. Neurol Med Chir (Tokyo) 1992; 32: 5-9
70. Ogawa A, Kameyama M, Muraishi K, et al. Cerebral blood flow and metabolism following superficial temporal artery to superior cerebellar artery bypass for vertebrobasilar occlusive disease. J Neurosurg 1992; 76: 955-60
71. Powers WJ, Grubb Jr RL, Raichle ME. Clinical results of extracranial-intracranial bypass surgery in patients with hemodynamic cerebrovascular disease. J Neurosurg 1989; 70: 61-7
72. Tenjin H, Ueda S, Mizukawa N, et al. Positron emission tomographic measurement of acute hemodynamic changes in primate middle cerebral artery occlusion. Neurol Med Chir (Tokyo) 1992; 32: 805-10
73. Pappata S, Fiorelli M, Rommel T, et al. PET study of changes in local brain hemodynamics and oxygen metabolism after unilateral middle cerebral artery occlusion in baboons. J Cereb Blood Flow Metab 1993; 13: 416-24

74. Heiss W-D, Graf R, Wienhard K, et al. Dynamic penumbra demonstrated by sequential multitracer PET after middle cerebral artery occlusion in cats. J Cereb Blood Flow Metab 1994; 14: 892-902
75. Heiss W-D, Wienhard K, Graf R, et al. High-resolution PET in cats: application of a clinical camera to experimental studies. J Nucl Med 1995; 36: 493-8
76. Young AR, Touzani O, Baron J-C, et al. To reperfuse or not to reperfuse?: Quantitative infarct volumes after middle cerebral artery occlusion in the baboon [abstract]. J Cereb Blood Flow Metab 1995; 15 Suppl. 1: S72
77. Touzani O, Young AR, Derlon J-M, et al. Sequential studies of severely hypometabolic tissue volumes after permanent middle cerebral artery occlusion: a positron emission tomographic investigation in anesthetized baboons. Stroke 1995; 26: 2112-9
78. Heiss W-D, Graf R, Löttgen J, et al. Repeat positron emission tomographic studies in transient middle cerebral artery occlusion in cats: residual perfusion and efficacy of postischemic reperfusion. J Cereb Blood Flow Metab 1997; 17: 388-400
79. Hayakawa T, Waltz AG. Changes of epidural pressures after experimental occlusion of middle cerebral artery in cats: relationship to severity of neurologic deficits, sizes of infarcts, and anesthesia. J Neurol Sci 1975; 26: 319-33
80. Young AR, Sette G, Touzani O, et al. Relationships between high oxygen extraction fraction in the acute stage and final infarction in reversible middle cerebral artery occlusion: an investigation in anesthetized baboons with positron emission tomography. J Cereb Blood Flow Metab 1996; 16: 1176-88
81. Warach S, Boska M, Welch KMA. Pitfalls and potential of clinical diffusion-weighted MR imaging in acute stroke. Stroke 1997; 28: 481-2
82. Moseley ME, Cohen Y, Mintorovitch J, et al. Early detection of regional cerebral ischemia in cats: comparison of diffusion- and T2-weighted MRI and spectroscopy. Magn Reson Med 1990; 14: 330-46
83. Warach S. Diffusion-weighted imaging. In: Moskowitz MA, Caplan LR, editors. Cerebrovascular diseases. Boston: Butterworth-Heinemann, 1995: 451-62
84. Mintorovitch J, Moseley ME, Chileuitt L, et al. Comparison of diffusion- and T2-weighted MRI for the early detection of cerebral ischemia and reperfusion in rats. Magn Reson Med 1991; 18: 39-50
85. Hoehn-Berlage M, Norris DG, Kohno K, et al. Evolution of regional changes in apparent diffusion coefficient during focal ischemia of rat brain: the relationship of quantitative diffusion NMR imaging to reduction in cerebral blood flow and metabolic disturbances. J Cereb Blood Flow Metab 1995; 15: 1002-11
86. Hossmann K-A, Hoehn-Berlage M. Diffusion and perfusion MR imaging of cerebral ischemia. Cerebrovasc Brain Metab Rev 1995; 7: 187-217
87. Rother J, de Crespigny AJ, D'Arceuil H, et al. Recovery of apparent diffusion coefficient after ischemia-induced spreading depression relates to cerebral perfusion gradient. Stroke 1996; 27: 980-6
88. Mintorovitch J, Chen J, Tsuura M, et al. Delayed neuronal death predicted by early diffusion-weighted hyperintensity in temporary focal ischemia in a rat model [abstract]. 11th Annual Meeting of the Society of Magnetic Resonance in Medicine; 1992 Aug 8-14; Berlin, 1805
89. Minematsu K, Li L, Fisher M, et al. Diffusion-weighted magnetic resonance imaging: rapid and quantitative detection of focal brain ischemia. Neurology 1992; 42: 235-40
90. Hasegawa Y, Fisher M, Latour LL, et al. MRI diffusion mapping of reversible and irreversible ischemic injury in focal brain ischemia. Neurology 1994; 44: 1484-90
91. Miyabe M, Mori S, van Zijl PC, et al. Correlation of the average water diffusion constant with cerebral blood flow and ischemic damage after transient middle cerebral artery occlusion in cats. J Cereb Blood Flow Metab 1996; 16: 881-91
92. Hasegawa Y, Latour LL, Formato JE, et al. Spreading waves of a reduced diffusion coefficient of water in normal and ischemic rat brain. J Cereb Blood Flow Metab 1995; 15: 179-87
93. Takano K, Latour LL, Formato JE, et al. The role of spreading depression in focal ischemia evaluated by diffusion mapping. Ann Neurol 1996; 39: 308-18
94. Lo EH, Matsumoto K, Pierce AR, et al. Pharmacologic reversal of acute changes in diffusion-weighted magnetic resonance imaging in focal cerebral ischemia. J Cereb Blood Flow Metab 1994; 14: 597-603
95. Hall WL, Benveniste H, Hedlund LW, et al. A new *in vivo* method for quantitative analysis of stroke lesions using diffusion-weighted magnetic resonance microscopy. Neuroimage 1996; 3: 158-66
96. Busch E, Gyngell ML, Eis M, et al. Potassium-induced cortical spreading depressions during focal cerebral ischemia in rats: contribution to lesion growth assessed by diffusion-weighted NMR and biochemical imaging. J Cereb Blood Flow Metab 1996; 16: 1090-9
97. Minematsu K, Fisher M, Davis MA, et al. Effects of a novel NMDA antagonist on experimental stroke rapidly and quantitatively assessed by diffusion-weighted MRI. Neurology 1993; 43: 397-403
98. Warach S, Moseley M, Sorensen AG, et al. Time course of diffusion imaging abnormalities in human stroke. Stroke 1996; 27: 1254-5
99. Welch KMA, Levine SR, Chopp M, et al. Time course of diffusion imaging abnormalities in human stroke. Stroke 1996; 27: 1255-6
100. Ulug AM, Beauchamp N, Bryan RN, et al. Absolute quantitation of diffusion constants in human stroke. Stroke 1997; 28: 483-90
101. Edelman RR, Warach S. Magnetic resonance imaging. N Engl J Med 1993; 328: 785-91
102. Warach S, Chien D, Li W, et al. Fast magnetic resonance diffusion-weighted imaging of acute human stroke. Neurology 1992; 42: 1717-23
103. Le Bihan D, Turner R, Douek P, et al. Diffusion MR imaging: clinical applications. Am J Roentgenol 1992; 159: 591-9

104. Chien D, Kwong KK, Gress DR, et al. MR diffusion imaging of cerebral infarction in humans. AJNR Am J Neuroradiol 1992; 13: 1097-102
105. Warach S, Gaa J, Siewert B, et al. Acute human stroke studied by whole brain echo planar diffusion-weighted magnetic resonance imaging. Ann Neurol 1995; 37: 231-41
106. Marks MP, de Crespigny A, Lentz D, et al. Acute and chronic stroke: navigated spin-echo diffusion-weighted MR imaging. Radiology 1996; 199: 403-8
107. Welch KM, Windham J, Knight RA, et al. A model to predict the histopathology of human stroke using diffusion and T2-weighted magnetic resonance imaging. Stroke 1995; 26: 1983-9
108. Warach S, Benfield A, Schlaug G, et al. Reduction of lesion volume in human stroke by citicoline detected by diffusion-weighted magnetic resonance imaging: pilot study [abstract]. Ann Neurol 1996; 40: 527
109. Hsu CY. Criteria for valid preclinical trials using animal stroke models. Stroke 1993; 24: 633-6
110. Ringelstein EB, Biniek R, Weiller C, et al. Type and extent of hemispheric brain infarctions and clinical outcome in early and delayed middle cerebral artery recanalization. Neurology 1992; 42: 289-98
111. Del Zoppo GJ. Thrombolytic therapy in acute stroke: recent experience. Cerebrovasc Dis 1993; 3: 256-63
112. Müller-Küppers M, Brandt T, von Kummer R, et al. Late clinical outcome of survivors of basilar artery occlusion and thrombolytic therapy [abstract]. Stroke 1994; 25: 256
113. Koudstaal PJ, Stibbe J, Vermeulen M. Fatal ischaemic brain oedema after early thrombolysis with tissue plasminogen activator in acute stroke. BMJ 1988; 297: 1571-4
114. Wolpert SM, Bruckmann H, Greenlee R, et al. Neuroradiologic evaluation of patients with acute stroke treated with recombinant tissue plasminogen activator. AJNR Am J Neuroradiol 1993; 14: 3-13
115. Hacke W, Stingele R, Steiner T, et al. Critical care of acute ischemic stroke. Intensive Care Med 1995; 21: 856-62
116. Heiss W-D, Grond M, Thiel A, et al. Tissue at risk of infarction rescued by early reperfusion: a positron emission tomography study in systemic recombinant tissue plasminogen activator thrombolysis of acute stroke. J Cereb Blood Flow Metab 1998; 18: 1298-1307
117. Ginsberg MD. The concept of the therapeutic window: a synthesis of critical issues. In: Moskowitz MA, Caplan LR, editors. Cerebrovascular diseases. Boston: Butterworth-Heinemann, 1995: 331-51
118. Baron JC, von Kummer R, del Zoppo GJ. Treatment of acute ischemic stroke: challenging the concept of a rigid and universal time window. Stroke 1995; 26: 2219-21
119. Garcia JH, Lassen NA, Weiller C, et al. Ischemic stroke and incomplete infarction. Stroke 1996; 27: 761-5
120. Fisher M, Garcia JH. Evolving stroke and the ischemic penumbra. Neurology 1996; 47: 884-8
121. Major ongoing stroke trials. Stroke 1994; 25: 541-5
122. Mohr JP, Orgogozo JM, Harrison MJG, et al. Meta-analysis of oral nimodipine trials in acute ischemic stroke. Cerebrovasc Dis 1994; 4: 197-203
123. Heiss W-D, Holthoff V, Hartmann-Klosterkötter U, et al. Nimodipine improves glucose metabolism after stroke. Stroke 1990; 21 Suppl. 1: I158-9
124. Huber M, Kittner B, Hojer C, et al. Effect of propentofylline on regional cerebral glucose metabolism in acute ischemic stroke. J Cereb Blood Flow Metab 1993; 13: 526-30

Correspondence: Prof. *Wolf-Dieter Heiss*, Max-Planck-Institut für neurologische Forschung, Gleueler Strasse 50, D-50931 Cologne, Germany.

Drug Therapy for Acute Ischaemic Stroke

Risks versus Benefits

Richard I. Lindley

Department of Clinical Neurosciences, University of Edinburgh, Bramwell Dott Building, Western General Hospital, Edinburgh, Scotland

Stroke is common, frequently disabling and often fatal.[1,2] Therapeutic nihilism has dominated stroke medicine for decades but this attitude can no longer be justified.[3] Recent trials have provided evidence for the balance of the risks and benefits associated with a variety of drugs. In this review, the systematic assessment of patients with suspected stroke is described, and the roles of the new drug treatments in the light of recent studies are discussed.

Often the question is asked of why we have many treatments for acute myocardial infarction (AMI) and very little to offer the patient with acute stroke. The answer to this question is complex but can probably be explained by a few simple differences between stroke medicine and short term coronary care: the stroke syndrome is far more heterogeneous; until recently stroke units were few in number; and, patients with stroke are much older than those with AMI. Until computerised tomographic (CT) scanning was widely available we were unable to reliably distinguish ischaemic stroke from primary intracerebral haemorrhage. The inability to diagnose the underlying pathology of stroke correctly severely compromised early trials of antithrombotic therapy and thrombolytic therapy for acute stroke. Finally, stroke disease is primarily a disease of the elderly and the elderly dysphasic stroke patient does not attract the attention the same sort of attention as a 40-year-old patient who survives an AMI.

The series of 'mega-trials' for AMI which emerged in the past decade have taught physicians many lessons.[4] First and foremost is the surprisingly large number of patients that need to be randomised to provide really reliable evidence of the balance of risks and benefits of treatments with only moderate effects.[5] Expert opinion, the mainstay of medical education since the time of Hippocrates, has many advantages but unfortunately is hopeless if the expert turns out to be wrong.[6,7] In practical terms there are 2 main requirements for the assessment of new treatments: first, large numbers of patients need to be randomised (to reduce random error as individuals are so different from each other); and secondly, true random allocation and blinded assessment eliminates a systematic bias.[5]

1. Short Term Stroke Treatment: A Step-Wise Approach

The best clinical units are those where attention to detail is combined with a simple but systematic approach to a clinical problem. Such an approach is vital for the rational use of drugs for patients in the acute phase of stroke. Figure 1 illustrates the simple steps to be taken when assessing a patient with suspected stroke. In the following section these simple questions illustrating the role of drug therapy at each point will be described in more detail.

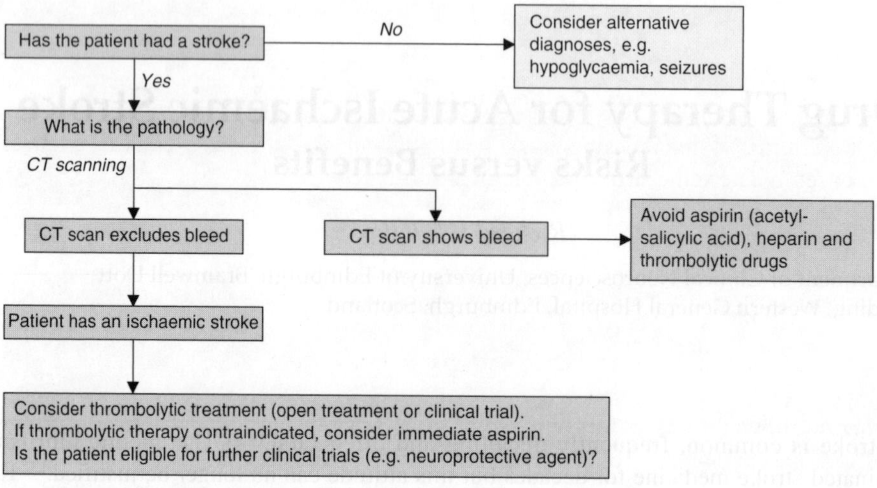

Fig. 1. A simple pathway for stroke care. **CT** = computerised tomography.

1.1 Is it a Stroke?

Bedside diagnosis is surprisingly accurate if care is taken to get a third party history. The telephone is a powerful tool in obtaining diagnostic information. Key parts of the history include questioning the patient (or relative, or carer) about stroke risk factors and the onset of symptoms. Stroke is usually defined as a sudden onset of focal (or global) loss of cerebral function with symptoms lasting more than 24 hours (or leading to death) with a presumed vascular cause.[8]

Whilst this definition is useful for epidemiology it is less useful in the emergency room when 'time is brain'. If we wait 24 hours to check if it really is a stroke we miss the therapeutic window! A more pragmatic definition for acute stroke care would not include the 24-hour time limit but an acceptance that symptoms that fail to resolve within an hour or two are likely to represent a stroke if left untreated, and thus urgent assessment should proceed. A major aim of acute stroke treatment is to convert a potentially irreversible event (the stroke) into a transient event (a transient ischaemic attack; TIA).

Once we are convinced we are dealing with an acute cerebral vascular event the next step is to identify the underlying stroke pathology.

1.2 What is the Stroke Pathology?

Most strokes are due to cerebral infarction[1] and, whilst clinical scoring systems can help predict infarct from haemorrhage,[9-11] the gold standard investigation remains CT scanning. Bleeding due to primary intracerebral haemorrhage is immediately visible on the CT scan; thus, CT scanning can exclude a bleed. As subsequent treatment depends on the pathology of the stroke, an early CT scan is vital in the short term management of stroke. The longer a CT scan is delayed the less certain the initial pathology, as bleeding into a cerebral infarct can occur, mimicking a primary intracerebral haemorrhage.[12] This implies that if the CT scan is delayed (e.g. 24 hours after the onset of stroke symptoms) and the scan appearance is that of a primary intracerebral haemorrhage, there could be uncertainty about the initial stroke pathology. Such an appearance may represent a primary intracerebral haemorrhage, or massive haemorrhagic transformation of cerebral infarction. It is also illogical to delay CT scanning until such time that the cerebral infarct is visible as the main rationale of treatment is to prevent such infarction. The main message must be to perform CT scanning as early as possible after stroke onset to determine stroke pathological sub-type.

1.3 What Should be Done Immediately?

After diagnosing the stroke and excluding a primary intracerebral haemorrhage we are now in a position to consider urgent treatment. At this stage patients (and their relatives and carers) need information and explanation, so they should be told the likely diagnosis. During the preceding clinical assessment a bedside swallow assessment should be performed to assess whether swallowing is safe. Not only is this good practice but it allows sensible prescribing of subsequent treatment.

1.4 The Drug Treatment of Ischaemic Stroke

1.4.1 Thrombolytic Therapy

Ischaemic stroke is due to occluded cerebral (or extracranial) arteries and a rational treatment is one which recanalises the occluded vessels and protects the ischaemic brain until full revascularisation can occur.

Thrombolytic therapy, which revolutionised AMI treatment, has now been evaluated in patients with acute ischaemic stroke. As the trials have been rather small, the results from individual studies are prone to false positive and false negative results.

To try and reduce the effects of random error the risks and benefits of treatment derived from a recent meta-analysis published electronically in the Cochrane library, and in a recent paper, will be discussed.[13,14]

The totality of the evidence suggests that whilst very early treatment can improve long term outcome, there are substantial early risks of cerebral haemorrhage. Only 12 trials, including a total of 3435 patients, were identified. Brain imaging prior to randomisation was mandatory in all these studies to exclude strokes due to primary intracerebral haemorrhage and drug treatment was given using the intravenous route. Three trials used urokinase, four trials used streptokinase and five trials used a tissue plasminogen activator (t-PA). All but the Multicentre Acute Stroke Trial – Italy Group[15] trial were placebo controlled. Although five trials had no age limit, six trials excluded those over 80 years of age and one study excluded those over 85 years.

One interesting point to note was the very large difference in case-fatality between some of trials (as observed in the placebo group). This suggests that the studies included rather different types of populations and as a consequence the results of the overview may not be generalisable.

Overall, allocation to thrombolytic therapy was associated with a statistically significant absolute reduction of 6.5% in longer term poor outcome (i.e. dead or dependent 3 to 6 months after stroke). This absolute reduction can be stated as about 65 extra patients alive and independent, per 1000 treated with thrombolytic therapy (95% confidence interval 28 to 107). This substantial treatment effect can be compared with the effect of streptokinase in AMI which had a treatment effect of 28 deaths prevented per 1000 patients treated in the ISIS-2[4] trial.

However, this substantial benefit with drug treatment was associated with significant risks.[14] There was an early excess of deaths (about 90 extra early deaths per 1000 treated). In addition, there was a substantial early hazard due to cerebral haemorrhage. There were an extra 70 symptomatic cerebral bleeds, of which about 50 were fatal per 1000 treated. Interestingly, the excess of deaths in the thrombolytic treatment groups was less marked at the end of the trial follow-up suggesting that thrombolytic therapy tends to have a net effect of accelerating death due to stroke. Of course, we simply do not know whether the patients who die because of complications of thrombolytic therapy were the ones who would have died if untreated.

Other important data to emerge from this overview included the evidence that the delay in treatment is important. The excess of deaths seemed to disappear if analysis was restricted to those randomised within 3 hours of stroke onset. Unfortunately, the systematic review included too few patients to provide reliable evidence of statistically significant differences in the treatment effects of the different types of thrombolytic agent, especially if very early treatment alone was considered (within 3 hours of onset of symptoms).

A word of caution is needed in the interpretation of these data as there was significant heterogeneity between the studies. This implies that the studies were very different from each other and can indicate that some of the trials were unusually optimistic or pessimistic in the individual estimates of treatment effects.

Alternatively, the heterogeneity may be the result of significant methodological differences and thus the one positive publication that was significant in its own right needs particular scrutiny. This publication, from the National Institute of Neurological Disorders and Stroke rt-PA Stroke Study Group (NINDS), reported the combined results from two very similar studies of very early administration of the recombinant t-PA alteplase.[16] Close inspection of the NINDS paper will help guide clinicians in their decision to use a t-PA (table I), but the decision to license alteplase for this indication has been controversial.[18]

The possibility that the positive results from these two trials were due to chance have been dismissed by some[18] but cannot be excluded, especially in view of the other less promising results. To help get around these difficulties, well organised stroke centres should have very strict protocols for the emergency use of alteplase for highly selected patients. Participation in further random-

Table I. Suggested checklist for hospital units wishing to offer emergency treatment with tissue plasminogen activator (t-PA) for patients with acute ischaemic stroke

Have you a well organised hospital stroke service?
Have you a mechanism to quickly identify patients with stroke in the emergency room?
Can you 'fast-track' patients to the computerised tomographic scanner?
Have you got intensive care back up facilities?
Patient selection for emergency treatment with t-PA
Patient (or appropriate delegate) consents to treatment?
Clear history of the time of onset of symptoms of acute stroke?
Computerised tomographic scan has excluded intracerebral haemorrhage?
Treatment can be started within 3 hours of onset of stroke symptoms?
Stroke symptoms not improving rapidly (i.e. unlikely to be a transient ischaemic attack?)
No contraindications to thrombolytic therapy such as:
No recent head trauma?
No surgery within previous 14 days?
No evidence of gastrointestinal haemorrhage or haematuria in previous 21 days?
Systolic blood pressure <185mm Hg; diastolic pressure <110mm Hg?
No arterial puncture at a noncompressible site within previous 7 days?
No coagulopathy, e.g. advanced liver disease
No concurrent warfarin or heparin treatment (unless normal clotting studies)?
Mimics of severe stroke excluded (seizures[17] and hypoglycaemia)?

ised trials of thrombolytic therapy versus placebo should also be encouraged.

It must be noted that evidence from randomised controlled trials involving over 17 000 patients was required to convince doctors that thrombolytic therapy was effective for patients with AMI.[4,19] It is likely that a larger study than the NINDS trial will be needed to convince doctors that the risks of thrombolytic therapy are worth the later benefits for acute ischaemic stroke. Meta-analysis may convince some but not all. The results of the thrombolytic trials to date raise more questions (table II) than answers and these uncertainties will only be resolved by further trials. Urgent research is needed to develop safer thrombolytic agents (or more focused use of available agents). Many thousands more patients may need to be randomised to provide really reliable data on the balance of risks and benefits, but this is not an unreasonable request. Do we really want to base our treatment of the next few million strokes on a trial of a few hundred patients?

Table II. Remaining uncertainties about thrombolytic therapy for acute ischaemic stroke

What is the precise time window?
Which thrombolytic agent is most beneficial?
What is the optimal dose?
Is the treatment of severe hypertension mandatory?
Are there any age limits to treatment?
Are very early computerised tomographic scan changes of ischaemia an absolute contraindication to treatment?
Who is at particular risk of intracerebral haemorrhage?
How precise are the treatment effects?
Should we avoid heparin treatment?
When is it safe/appropriate to start aspirin (acetylsalicylic acid)?

1.4.2 Antithrombotic Therapy

Following the publication of the International Stroke Trial[20] and the Chinese Acute Stroke Study,[21] we now have evidence from randomised controlled trials of the balance of risks and benefits of immediate antithrombotic therapy from about 20 000 patients for heparin and 40 000 patients for aspirin (acetylsalicylic acid). *In summary,* immediate aspirin can be safely recommended for most patients with ischaemic stroke but as yet there are no convincing data that immediate heparin has any net benefit.

1.4.3 Aspirin (Acetylsalicylic Acid)

Aspirin is a proven treatment for AMI and is now well established for the secondary prevention of vascular events for a wide variety of patients at high risk of vascular death.[4,22] In addition, meta-analysis has shown that aspirin can prevent deep vein thrombosis (a recognised complication of stroke).[23] It was therefore considered a promising treatment for acute ischaemic stroke.

The International Stroke Trial was a pragmatic, open randomised controlled trial that aimed to include a wide variety of patients with acute ischaemic stroke from a wide variety of hospitals in many countries. Trial procedures were simplified to facilitate participation in the study. The entry criteria were straightforward:

- a clinical diagnosis of stroke with onset of symptoms first noted within previous 48 hours
- no clear indication or contraindication for immediate aspirin or heparin
- uncertainty of the benefit of early antithrombotic treatment
- no evidence of intracerebral haemorrhage (CT scanning was strongly advised but not mandatory prior to randomisation).

Those allocated to immediate aspirin were prescribed aspirin in a dose of 300 mg/day and rectal aspirin was recommended if the patient was unable to swallow. Treatment was continued for 14 days (or hospital discharge if sooner). Treatment was not blinded, but efforts were made to blind the 6-month assessment of dependency for stroke survivors.

The entry criteria were identical in the Chinese Acute Stroke Study but the dose of aspirin was somewhat lower at 160mg/day and treatment was given in double-blind fashion for 1 month.

The results from these two very large studies were very similar (and support the notion that the blinded assessment of outcome in the International Stroke Trial was successful at reducing systematic bias). Individually, neither study was large enough in its own right to provide statistically significant results of the pre-specified analyses, due to the very modest benefit of aspirin.

However, in combining the aspirin results from both studies (and the small Multicentre Acute Stroke Trial – Italy Group trial[15]) there was a significant reduction in the rate of recurrent stroke and death in hospital of about 9 (SD = 3) per 1000 patients treated. About 11 (SD = 3) recurrent ischaemic strokes and deaths were prevented and there were about 2 (SD = 1) extra intracranial bleeds per 1000 patients treated. In addition, there was a significant reduction in those patients who died or were dependent at the end of trial follow-up with a benefit of about 11 (SD = 6) extra independent patients per 1000 treated. It should, however, be noted that there were some differences between the trials: patients in the Chinese Acute Stroke Study were more likely to have had a pre-randomisation CT scan and were of lower risk and younger in age.

There was no clear evidence of a relationship between the delay in starting treatment and treatment effect of aspirin; one explanation is that aspirin is merely acting as a secondary preventative agent with little influence on the initial area of infarction.

Treatment effects appeared similar across a large number of clinically identifiable subgroups. The concordance of the results suggests that aspirin is widely practicable but with a modest treatment effect. The paradox is that immediate aspirin may well prevent many more patients dying or becoming disabled following an acute stroke than thrombolytic therapy. This is because aspirin can be given to the vast majority of patients with ischaemic stroke while thrombolytic therapy is currently only applicable to highly selected patients. Hospital services need to be organised to ensure that this very cheap and simple treatment is not forgotten.

1.4.4 Heparin

Heparin has been used for decades for the treatment of stroke,[24-26] but despite a promising meta-analysis of earlier trials[27] the results of the International Stroke Trial do not support the routine use of heparin.[20] In the International Stroke Trial (see section 1.4.3) two doses of subcutaneous unfractionated heparin were tested: 5000U twice daily and 12 500U twice daily. Monitoring of the activated partial thromboplastin times was not mandatory and left to the discretion of the attending physician (treatment was not blinded). The rationale of using a fixed subcutaneous dose was to simplify the treatment, avoid the inevitable stop/start problems of intravenous treatment and not interfere with early rehabilitation.

The pre-specified analyses for the heparin groups of the International Stroke Trial were early mortality (deaths within 14 days of randomisation) and 6-month poor outcome (dead or dependency). At 14 days there were non-significantly fewer deaths in the heparin allocated patients (9 *vs* 9.3%). More deaths in the heparin group were due to intra- and extracranial bleeding (40 *vs* 18). At 6 months the proportion of dead or dependent patients were identical for the heparin and 'avoid heparin' groups at 62.9%.

These disappointing results hide a fascinating mix of risks and benefits as heparin significantly reduced the chance of early recurrent ischaemic stroke (2.9% for the heparin group versus 3.8% for the control) which was offset by an increase in haemorrhagic recurrent stroke (1.2 *vs* 0.4%). Both results were highly significant. In addition, heparin was associated with a significant excess of transfused or fatal extracranial bleeds mainly attributable to the 12 500U twice daily heparin regimen. Many clinicians are convinced that patients in atrial fibrillation must be anticoagulated immediately after the onset of ischaemic stroke yet the International Stroke Trial has shown that the reduction in recurrent ischaemic stroke is still offset by the increase in recurrent haemorrhagic stroke (table III).

Table III. Heparin is not beneficial for patients in atrial fibrillation and recent ischaemic stroke[a]

	Heparin (%) [n = 9716]	No heparin (%) [n = 9717]
Patients in sinus rhythm		
Recurrent ischaemic stroke	2.9	3.6*
Recurrent haemorrhagic stroke	1.1	0.4**
Total recurrent stroke	4.0	4
Death or nonfatal stroke	10.3	10.3
Patients in atrial fibrillation		
Recurrent ischaemic stroke	2.8	4.9***
Recurrent haemorrhagic stroke	2.1	0.4****
Total recurrent stroke	4.9	5.3
Death or nonfatal stroke	19.1	20.7

a This table summarises the risks and benefits of subcutaneous heparin for patients with ischaemic stroke subdivided by cardiac rhythm in the International Stroke Trial.[20] The figures refer to events within the 14-day allocated treatment period. It can be seen that patients in atrial fibrillation have a higher absolute risk of poor outcome compared to those in sinus rhythm. The significant reductions due to heparin in recurrent ischaemic strokes are offset by the risk of recurrent haemorrhagic strokes even for those in atrial fibrillation. This table is a subgroup analysis of the patients randomised in the International Stroke Trial.[20]

* 2p < 0.05; ** 2p < 0.01; *** 2p < 0.001; **** 2p < 0.00001.

Are there any data from the International Stroke Trial to suggest that certain subgroups may benefit from treatment? Unfortunately, close inspection of the many published subgroup analyses is not encouraging. In fact, there is evidence that those with severe strokes (e.g. those patients with a large cortical infarct or depressed consciousness level or a poor prognostic stroke) do particularly badly. This finding is consistent with the view that the larger the infarct, the greater the risk of haemorrhagic transformation of infarction. As only 5000 patients were randomised to the smaller heparin dose (5000U twice daily), there are insufficient data to reliably detect an additional small benefit of adding low dose subcutaneous heparin to aspirin for the early treatment of ischaemic stroke.

What does all this mean in routine clinical practice? Patients with no clear contraindication to aspirin should be given aspirin immediately after a CT scan has excluded a primary intracerebral haemorrhage. Routine use of heparin should be avoided unless required for another specific indication (e.g. pulmonary embolism or deep vein thrombosis). Patients in atrial fibrillation should be given aspirin for the first 2 weeks. At the end of 2 weeks of treatment clinicians should consider starting warfarin and stopping the aspirin if there are no contraindications to oral anticoagulation.

Low molecular weight heparin and heparinoids have not been tested in large enough studies to provide reliable data on effectiveness. The preliminary results of the randomised trial of danaparoid sodium (ORG-10172) in acute stroke were also disappointing.[28]

1.4.5 Neuroprotective Agents

The main focus of treatment for ischaemic stroke is to restore the normal vascular anatomy. Without an adequate blood supply, the brain will undergo infarction. During the early phase of ischaemia there is a therapeutic opportunity to halt or reverse the harmful influx of calcium into the cells, as well as to reduce (or antagonise) the release of the neurotoxic excitatory amino acids.[29,30] These treatment strategies, the so-called neuroprotective agents, may extend the time window for successful revascularisation and add to the benefits of antithrombotic and fibrinolytic agents. A detailed discussion is beyond the scope of this review but the reviews by Muir[29] and Dorman[30] offer a useful summary.

1.4.6 Other Treatments

Many other drugs have now been evaluated in patients with acute ischaemic stroke but none have shown a significant overall benefit. With few exceptions all the randomised controlled trials have been too small to reliably exclude a moderate beneficial treatment effect. Whilst phase I trials are vital to evaluate the safety of new drugs (or new indications for older drugs), they should not used to eliminate promising drugs merely because the results are rather disappointing. The play of chance overwhelms many treatment effects, and trials sponsored by pharmaceutical companies still tend to be too small, with a major risk of false positive or negative results. In addition, there is a real risk that promising neuroprotective drugs are being discarded too early in development.

Table IV. Treatments for acute stroke

Treatment	Comment
Aspirin (acetylsalicylic acid)	Beneficial
Unfractionated heparin	Risks outweigh benefits
Low molecular weight heparin	More trials needed
Danaparoid sodium (ORG-10172)	Await final results from TOAST but likely to be similar to heparin
Thrombolytic therapy	More trials needed, some centres use tissue plasminogen activators
Lubeluzole[31]	More trials needed
Intravenous magnesium[32]	More trials needed
Glycerol[33]	More trials needed (in certain subgroups)
Corticosteroids	More trials needed (in certain subgroups)
Mannitol	More trials needed (in certain subgroups)
Benzodiazepines	More trials needed
Ancrod[33]	More trials needed
Batroxobin[33]	More trials needed
Methylxanthines[33]	More trials needed
Epoprostenol (prostacyclin)	More trials needed
Calcium antagonists	More trials needed
Clomethiazole (chlormethiazole)	More trials needed
NMDA receptor antagonists	Can adverse effects be reduced?
Gangliosides[33]	Not worthwhile
Haemodilution[34]	Not worthwhile
Enlimomab (antileucocyte)	More studies needed (septicaemic complications too great in initial clinical trials)
Blood pressure manipulation	More studies needed
Blood glucose lowering[35]	Trials needed for hyperglycaemic patients

NMDA = *N*-demethyl-D-aspartate; **TOAST** = the randomised trial of danaparoid sodium (a heparinoid also known as ORG-10172) in acute stroke.

Table IV lists some promising drugs (or treatment strategies) which need to be evaluated further and also some treatments which are probably ineffective. Large phase III trials are planned for the neuroprotective agents lubeluzole, intravenous magnesium and benzodiazepines and the results are awaited with interest. Clinical classification of ischaemic stroke subtype has been shown to be feasible in the acute phase of stroke and this new methodology will enable trials to concentrate on important stroke subtypes. For example, glycerol or corticosteroids should be evaluated for patients with large hemispheric infarction as identified by the Total Anterior Circulation Infarct (TACI) subtype using the Oxfordshire Community Stroke Classification.[17]

Blood pressure lowering may be detrimental in the acute phase of stroke and more work is needed in this area.[36,37] Lowering of elevated glucose levels may be another metabolic strategy worth pursuing.[35]

2. The Future

We now have the trial methodology to test simple practicable treatments in tens of thousands of patients with acute ischaemic stroke; still, many more 'mega-trials' are needed to identify treatments with moderate benefits. Meta-analyses of small trials will help guide whether further trials are worthwhile and will summarise the world evidence in the absence of a single convincing study.[38] In addition, subtype classification of the heterogeneous group of patients with cerebral infarction will allow focused treatment targeted to the presumed underlying pathology.

It is very unlikely that there is a panacea for all types of ischaemic stroke (aspirin may the best agent in this regard), and thus logical combinations of treatment should be evaluated. For example, a 2 × 2 factorial design of a neuroprotector and thrombolytic drug seems a very worthwhile design.

Stroke physicians should ensure their local hospitals provide organised stroke services.[39] There is no doubt that stroke units will facilitate further research. Efforts to reduce the delay from stroke onset to medical attention are likely to be beneficial and will allow specialised units to consider thrombolytic therapy for highly selected patients.[40]

As we currently lack an ideal stroke treatment we must all encourage participation in acute stroke trials as part of our routine clinical practice. Only data from randomised controlled trials will change clinical practice for the better.

References

1. Bamford J, Sandercock P, Dennis M, et al . A prospective study of acute cerebrovascular disease in the community: the Oxfordshire Community Stroke Project 1981-86. 1. Methodology, demography and incident cases of first-ever stroke. J Neurol Neurosurg Psychiatry 1988; 51: 1373-80
2. Bamford J, Sandercock P, Dennis M, et al. A prospective study of acute cerebrovascular disease in the community: the Oxfordshire Community Stroke Project-1981-1986 2. Incidence, case fatality and overall outcome at one year of cerebral infarction, primary intracerebral haemorrhage and subarachnoid haemorrhage. J Neurol Neurosurg Psychiatry 1990; 53: 16-22
3. The European Ad Hoc Consensus Group. European strategies for early intervention in stroke: a report of an Ad Hoc Consensus Group Meeting. Cerebrovasc Dis 1996; 6: 315-24
4. ISIS-2 Collaborative Group. Randomised trial of intravenous streptokinase, oral aspirin, both, or neither among 17,187 cases of suspected acute myocardial infarction: ISIS-2. Lancet 1988; 2: 349-60
5. Yusuf S, Collins R, Peto R. Why do we need some large, simple randomised trials? Stat Med 1984; 3: 409-20
6. Sackett DL, Haynes RB, Tugwell P. Clinical epidemiology: a basic science for clinical medicine. Boston/Toronto: Little, Brown and Company, 1985
7. Antman EM, Lau J, Kupelnick B, et al. A comparison of results of meta-analysis of randomized control trials and recommendations of clinical experts. JAMA 1992; 268: 240-8
8. Hatano S. Experience from a multicentre stroke register: a preliminary report. Bull World Heath Organ 1976; 54: 541-53
9. Allen CMC. Clinical diagnosis of the acute stroke syndrome. Q J Med 1983; 52: 515-23
10. Sandercock PAG, Allen CMC, Corston RN, et al. Clinical diagnosis of intracranial haemorrhage using Guy's Hospital score. BMJ 1985; 291: 1675-7
11. Poungvarin N, Viriyavejakul A, Komontri C. Siriraj stroke score and validation study to distinguish supratentorial intracerebral haemorrhage from infarction. BMJ 1991; 302: 1565-7
12. Bogousslavsky J, Regli F, Uske A, et al. Early spontaneous hematoma in cerebral infarct: is primary cerebral hemorrhage overdiagnosed? Neurology 1991; 41: 837-40
13. Wardlaw JM, Yamaguchi T, del Zoppo G, et al. Thrombolytic therapy versus control in acute ischaemic stroke. Stroke module of the Cochrane database of systematic reviews [updated 4 Mar 1997]. Available in The Cochrane Library [database on disk and CDROM]. The Cochrane Collaboration; Issue 2. Oxford: update software, 1997
14. Wardlaw JM, Warlow CP, Counsell C. Systematic review of evidence on thrombolytic therapy for acute ischaemic stroke. Lancet 1997; 350: 607-14
15. Multicentre Acute Stroke Trial - Italy (MAST-I) Group. Randomised controlled trial of streptokinase, aspirin, and combination of both in treatment of acute ischaemic stroke. Lancet 1995; 346: 1509-14
16. The National Institute of Neurological Disorders and Stroke rt-PA Stroke Study Group. Tissue plasminogen activator for acute ischemic stroke. N Engl J Med 1995; 333: 1581-7

17. Bamford J, Sandercock P, Dennis M, et al. Classification and natural history of clinically identifiable subtypes of cerebral infarction. Lancet 1991; 337: 1521-6
18. Caplan LR, Mohr JP, Kistler JP, et al. Clinical debate: should thrombolytic therapy be the first-line treatment for acute ischaemic stroke? N Engl J Med 1997; 337: 1309-13
19. Collins R, Julian D. British Heart Foundation surveys (1987 and 1989) of United Kingdom treatment policies for acute myocardial infarction. Br Heart J 1991; 66: 250-5
20. International Stroke Trial Collaborative Group. The International Stroke Trial (IST): a randomised trial of aspirin, subcutaneous heparin, both, or neither among 19435 patients with acute ischaemic stroke. Lancet 1997; 349: 1569-81
21. CAST (Chinse Acute Stroke Trial) Collaborative Group. CAST: randomised placebo-controlled trial of early aspirin use in 20 000 patients with acute ischaemic stroke. Lancet 1997; 349: 1641-9
22. Antiplatelet Trialists' Collaboration. Collaborative overview of randomised trials of antiplatelet treatment. Pt I: prevention of death, myocardial infarction and stroke by prolonged antiplatelet therapy in various categories of patients. BMJ 1994; 308: 81-106
23. Antiplatelet Trialists' Collaboration. Collaborative overview of randomised trials of antiplatelet therapy-III: reduction in venous thrombosis and pulmonary embolism by antiplatelet prophylaxis among surgical and medical patients. BMJ 1994; 308: 235-46
24. Jorpes JE. Heparin: a mucopolysaccharide and an active antithrombotic drug. Circulation 1959; 19: 87-91
25. Marsh EE, Adams HP, Biller J, et al. Use of antithrombotic drugs in the treatment of acute ischaemic stroke. A survey of neurologists in practice in the United States. Neurology 1989; 39: 1631-4
26. Lindley RI, Amayo EO, Marshall J, et al. Acute stroke treatment in UK hospitals: the Stroke Association survey of consultant opinion. J R Coll Physicians Lond 1995; 29: 479-84
27. Sandercock PAG, van den Belt AGM, Lindley RI, et al. Antithrombotic therapy in acute ischaemic stroke: an overview of the completed randomised trials. J Neurol Neurosurg Psychiatry 1993; 56: 17-25
28. The Publications Committee for the Trial of ORG-10172 in Acute Stroke Treatment (TOAST) Investigators. Low molecular weight heparinoid, ORG 10172 (danaparoid), and outcome after acute ischaemic stroke: a randomised controlled trial.JAMA 1998; 279: 1265-72
29. Muir KW. Lees KR. Clinical experience with excitatory amino acid antagonist drugs. Stroke 1995; 26: 503-13
30. Dorman P, Sandercock P. Design considerations in trials of neuroprotective therapy. Stroke 1996; 27: 1507-15
31. Diener HC, Hacke W, Hennerici M, et al. Lubeluzole in acute ischemic stroke: s double-blind, placebo-controlled Phase II Trial. Stroke 1996; 27: 76-81
32. Muir KW, Lees KR. A randomized, double-blind, placebo-controlled pilot trial of intravenous magnesium sulfate in acute stroke. Stroke 1995; 26: 1183-8
33. Stroke Module of the Cochrane Database of Systematic Reviews: (update software: available in the Cochrane Library). Oxford: Update Software, 1997 (database on disk and CDROM)
34. Asplund K. Hemodilution in acute stroke. Cerebrovasc Dis 1991; 1 Suppl. 1: 129-38
35. Weir CJ, Murray GD, Dyker AG, et al. Is hyperglycaemia an independent predictor of poor outcome after acute stroke? Results of a long term follow up study. BMJ 1997; 314: 1303-6
36. Wahlgren NG, McMahon DG, de Kayser J, et al. Intravenous Nimodipine West European Stroke Trial (INWEST) of nimodipine in the treatment of acute ischaemic stroke. Cerebrovasc Dis 1994; 4: 204-10
37. Phillips SJ. Pathophysiology and management of hypertension in acute ischemic stroke. Hypertension 1994; 23: 131-6
38. Counsell C, Warlow C, Sandercock P, et al. The Cochrane Collaboration Stroke Review Group: meeting the need for systematic reviews in stroke care. Stroke 1995; 26: 498-502
39. Stroke Unit Trialists' Collaboration. Collaborative systematic review of the randomised trials of organised inpatient (stroke unit) care after stroke. BMJ 1997; 314: 1151-9
40. Alberts MJ, Perry A, Dawson DV, et al. Effects of public and professional education on reducing the delay in presentation and referral of stroke patients. Stroke 1992; 23: 352-6

Correspondence: Dr *Richard I. Lindley*, Senior Lecturer, Department of Clinical Neurosciences, University of Edinburgh, Bramwell Dott Building, Western General Hospital, Edinburgh EH4 2XU, Scotland.
E-mail: ril@skull.dcn.ed.ac.uk

Recently Developed Neuroprotective Therapies for Acute Stroke

A Qualitative Systematic Review of Clinical Trials*

Paul J. Dorman, Carl E. Counsell and *Peter A.G. Sandercock*

Neurosciences Trials Unit, Department of Clinical Neurosciences, University of Edinburgh, Western General Hospital, Edinburgh, Scotland

Each year there are, in the US and European Union combined, approximately 1 million patients who have an acute stroke.[1] Stroke is not only the third most common cause of death in most developed countries, but is also the commonest cause of severe disability in the UK.[2] An effective and widely applicable medical treatment for acute stroke would have an enormous public health impact but, as yet, no such treatment has been found.[3]

Early interest in acute ischaemic stroke therapy focused on whether neurological outcomes might be improved by improving blood flow. Antithrombotic, thrombolytic and haemorrheological treatments were amongst the first approaches to be tested in randomised controlled trials.[4]

Increased understanding of the pathophysiological consequences of stroke and, in particular, the notion of an 'ischaemic penumbra' (see section 3.1) in acute ischaemic stroke has led to the development of a large number of new treatments. These treatments act at different stages of the pathophysiological cascade that begins with vessel occlusion (or rupture) and leads first to cellular ischaemia and finally to neuronal death.

1. Aims of the Review

Many pharmaceutical companies are actively developing neuroprotective compounds for use in humans. Not surprisingly, many clinicians interested in stroke are somewhat overwhelmed by the welter of information from these numerous trials. Available reviews of this area have focused on only certain neuroprotective agents [5,6] rather than giving an overview of all aspects of neuroprotection. This review therefore aims to:

(i) Briefly review the major cellular mechanisms that are thought to lead to neuronal cell death in acute ischaemic or haemorrhagic stroke.

(ii) Classify the agents currently in clinical development into broad groups on the basis of their proposed pharmacological effect.

(iii) Systematically identify and describe as many as possible of the completed, ongoing and planned randomised controlled trials evaluating the effect of the newer agents on clinical outcomes in stroke patients.

* This article is reprinted unchanged from the original version, which was published in June 1996.

(iv) Summarise and cite published quantitative systematic reviews of the 'older' agents, or reviews of these agents registered with the Stroke Review Group of the Cochrane Collaboration (see section 2.2).[7] We felt it unnecessary to duplicate detailed meta-analyses of agents where a significant amount of information from randomised controlled trials has already been or is in the process of being summarised.

We have restricted the scope of this review to randomised controlled trials evaluating agents for the treatment of patients with acute ischaemic or haemorrhagic stroke. We have deliberately excluded clinical trials in patients with subarachnoid haemorrhage or head injury as these are qualitatively different conditions.

2. Methods

2.1 Definition of Neuroprotective Therapy

For the purpose of this review we define a neuroprotective agent as one that aims to prevent neuronal death by inhibiting one or more of the pathophysiological steps in the processes that follow occlusion (or rupture) of a cerebral artery. This review will therefore not examine agents that act primarily to restore or improve blood flow (e.g. thrombolysis).

2.2 Methods for Identification of Studies for Inclusion

Relevant published and unpublished data from randomised controlled trials of neuroprotective therapy in acute stroke were identified from three sources:

- the Cochrane Collaboration Stroke Review Group's register of randomised controlled trials[7]
- additional bibliographic searching of reference lists of original research or review articles
- personal communications with the pharmaceutical companies known to be developing neuroprotective agents.

The Cochrane Collaboration Stroke Review Group's register has been assembled using a variety of search strategies including: (i) computerised bibliographic searching of the MEDLINE database from 1966 to the present (using a search strategy validated against hand searching); (ii) systematic hand searching of the 21 English language and five Japanese journals and the proceedings of more than 40 conferences related to stroke; (iii) searching bibliographies of reviews, trials, books and dissertations; (iv) personal contact with trialists; and (v) regular searches of the Ottawa Stroke Trials Registry.[8]

2.3 Data Extraction

Where possible the following data were extracted:

- the name of the agent
- the proposed mechanism of action
- the size of the clinical trial (and whether completed or underway)
- data on safety and efficacy, when available.

2.4 Data Synthesis

Formal quantitative meta-analysis of the results of the trials was not performed for two reasons. First, many of the published reports on new agents relate to pharmacology, pharmacokinetics and phase II clinical studies (e.g. dose-ranging studies) in which the outcomes measured were nonclinical. Secondly, as none of the novel neuroprotective agents has yet completed clinical development (or received a licence for use in acute stroke), the number of patients entered into controlled clinical trials, with clinically relevant measures of outcome (e.g. functional outcome), is very small. However, we did aim to describe the results of these trials qualitatively.

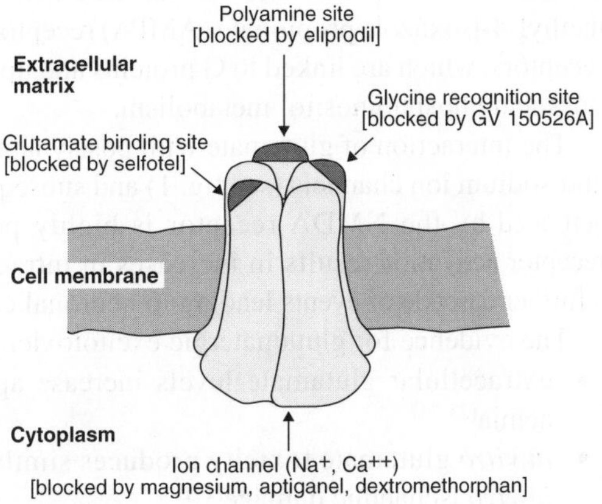

Fig. 1. Schematic representation of the *N*-methyl-D-aspartate receptor, showing the site of action of various agonists and antagonists.

3. What is the Pathophysiological Basis of Neuroprotection in Acute Cerebral Infarction?

3.1 The Ischaemic Penumbra

All neuroprotective agents are designed to 'rescue' ischaemically threatened, but potentially viable, tissue, the so-called 'ischaemic penumbra'. This penumbral tissue cannot be simply defined by its anatomical location. It is better defined as those neurons that suffer reduced blood supply, insufficient to maintain normal metabolic and functional activity, and are therefore affected by intermittent bioenergetic compromise, but are potentially viable if reperfused before irreversible cell damage has occurred.[9,10]

The dynamic, expanding nature of the altered metabolic and electrical activity of the penumbra has recently become clear.[11] Abnormal electrical activity plays a key role in spreading the ischaemic damage.[12] Permanent neuronal depolarisation occurs early on in the infarct core. Subsequently, waves of depolarisations spread into the peri-infarct tissue and adversely affect the survival of the penumbral tissue. This is because they increase the metabolic work (due to the increased energy demands of the activated ion exchange pumps)[13,14] without an adequate increase in blood supply. A cascade of interrelated biochemical and molecular processes are then thought to contribute to ischaemic cell damage. Similar penumbral tissue may exist in the brain around a primary intracerebral haemorrhage,[15,16] and many of the mechanisms leading to neuronal injury (see section 3.3) may be operative in both haemorrhagic and ischaemic stroke.

3.2 Excitatory Amino Acid (EAA) Release

Neuronal ischaemia results in the nonspecific release of excitatory amino acids (EAAs). These neurotransmitters activate specific receptor-operated ion channels; the subsequent ion fluxes then lead to membrane depolarisation. Glutamate is the best studied EAA involved in this process.[17,18] However, other neurotransmitters may also mediate ischaemic damage. Glycine [which functions as a co-agonist, potentiating the action of glutamate at the *N*-methyl-D-aspartate (NMDA) receptor (see fig. 1)] may be an important determinant of delayed neuronal injury.[19] Dopamine is also rapidly released at the onset of ischaemia, [19] although it is not clear whether this damages neurons.

Glutamate is the predominant excitatory neurotransmitter in the mammalian CNS. It is a mixed agonist that activates two main groups of receptor.[20] The first major group of receptors are linked to ionophores and include the NMDA (see fig. 1), kainate and α-amino-3-hydroxy-5-methyl-4-isoxazole propionate (AMPA) receptor types. The second group are the metabotropic receptors, which are linked to G proteins and upon activation induce changes in cyclic nucleotides and phosphoinositol metabolism.

The interaction of glutamate with postsynaptic receptors leads to the opening of calcium and sodium ion channels (see fig. 1) and subsequent membrane depolarisation. The ion channel activated by the NMDA receptor is highly permeable to calcium,[21] so excessive NMDA receptor activation results in increases in intracellular neuronal calcium to levels that initiate a further cascade of events leading to neuronal cell death.[22]

The evidence for glutamatergic excitotoxicity comes from several different areas:

- extracellular glutamate levels increase approximately 20-fold in acute cerebral ischaemia[23,24]
- *in vitro* glutamate toxicity produces similar histological appearances to that seen with *in vivo* ischaemic damage[25]
- the magnitude of the increase in glutamate levels correlates well with infarct volume[23]
- pharmacological inhibition of the glutamatergic system consistently reduces infarct volume in experimental models of focal ischaemia.[26]

This latter effect seems reproducible across many studies in different experimental models, in different animal species, and across a variety of different agents acting on the glutamatergic system in slightly different ways.[26,27]

Nitric oxide (NO, previously known as endothelium-derived relaxing factor) is synthesised by neuronal and glial tissue. The role of NO in cerebral ischaemia is not clear.[28] In ischaemic conditions, glutamatergic activity may lead to the generation of inducible NO synthetase. This may have adverse effects, as in the absence of L-arginine (the precursor of NO) it may generate neurotoxic superoxides and hydrogen peroxide.[29] However, experimental manipulation of the NO system in animal models of ischaemic stroke has produced conflicting results;[29] thus, it is difficult to predict the effect of this class of agent in humans.

3.3 What is the Final Common Pathway of Ischaemic Neuronal Injury?

Neuronal ischaemia, aggravated by inappropriate membrane depolarisations, results in progressive impairment of the energy-dependent membrane ion pumps. This leads to progressive derangement of cellular ion homeostasis: potassium leaks out of cells, sodium and water enter cells (which leads to cytotoxic oedema and cellular swelling) and calcium moves into cells.[30,31] Neuronal calcium homeostasis is further aggravated by both an activation of glutamate receptors, particularly the NMDA receptor, which leads to a massive calcium influx through receptor-activated calcium channels, and also by the release of sequestered intracellular calcium.[32]

Acidosis resulting from anaerobic glycolysis during sustained ischaemia contributes to tissue damage, oedema formation and independently interferes with mitochondrial function.[33] Numerous secondary processes occur thereafter to increase ischaemic neuronal damage, including: activation of proteolytic enzymes, phospholipases, protein kinases and generation of free radicals[34] from the breakdown of membrane phospholipids.

The onset of cerebral ischaemia is followed by the expression of genes whose activation may indicate inevitable cell death.[35] In addition, leucocytes attracted to the ischaemic area may potentiate brain injury by the production of cytotoxins, free radicals and phospholipases.[36] The temporal sequence and relative importance of each of these events remains unclear.

3.4 What is the Time Window for Neuroprotection in Humans?

The duration of the 'therapeutic window' for neuroprotective therapy following acute stroke in humans remains controversial. Experimental studies in a variety of animal models have failed to demonstrate significant protection if agents are administered more than 6 hours after the induction of ischaemia. However, stroke in humans differs fundamentally from that produced experimentally, and the relevance of the therapeutic window observed in animal studies must therefore be questioned.[37]

Observational studies using positron emission tomography (PET) have attempted indirectly to establish the duration of the therapeutic window in humans; tissue that is ischaemic, but still potentially viable, has been identified in the penumbra of the infarct more than 6 hours after symptom onset in patients with acute ischaemic stroke.[38,39] In 45 to 57% of cases of acute stroke, studied within 4 days of symptom onset, areas of tissue adjacent to the ischaemic core affected by 'misery perfusion' (characterised by an increased oxygen extraction fraction) were identified.[40] The fate of this tissue is unclear; ultimately it may survive and surround the infarct as a viable rim or alternatively it may simply become necrotic.[41] A recent study, using diffusion-weighted magnetic resonance imaging (MRI) showed that infarct lesion volumes continue to increase more than 12 hours after stroke onset.[42]

The demonstration that infarcts continue to increase more than 6 hours after onset and that there is potentially viable tissue at up to 4 days after stroke onset, raises the tantalising prospect that the therapeutic window for neuroprotection in humans may be significantly longer than that observed experimentally.

4. Systematic Review of the Randomised Controlled Trials of Neuroprotective Therapy in Acute Stroke

Reports of randomised controlled trials on 31 neuroprotective agents have been identified (although other agents are undergoing phase I and II evaluation, their progress is covered by confidentiality arrangements).

We have tried to produce a simple classification of the neuroprotective agents based on their presumed principal mode of action (table I). However, for several agents the mechanism of action in ischaemia is unknown (e.g. opioid receptor antagonists), and others have more than one potential mechanism of action, e.g. intravenous magnesium, calcium antagonists and NMDA receptor antagonists. In the latter case, we have tried to assign agents to the class relating to the mode of action that is presumed to be most important, although we accept this may be somewhat arbitrary.

4.1 Modulators of the EAA System

This class of agents consistently reduces infarct volume in a variety of animal models in a number of different species.[26,27] It may be subclassified into: (i) agents acting presynaptically on glutamate release; (ii) agents acting at the NMDA receptor itself; and (iii) agents that may exert postreceptor inhibition on glutamate-induced neuronal activation. The degree of neuro-

Table I. Classification system for neuroprotective therapies in stroke according to primary mechanism of action

Mechanism of action	Subclass	Example	Approximate no. patients enrolled in RCTs	
			completed or in progress	planned
Modulators of EAA system				
prereceptor effects[a]	Sodium channel modulators	Sibatragine	200	None
		Fos-phenytoin	100	600
	GABA agonist	Clomethiazole (chlormethiazole)	380	1350
	Barbiturate	Phenobarbital (phenobarbitone)	26	NA
	Adenosergic agent	Propentofylline	30	NA
NMDA receptor antagonists	Noncompetitive	Dextrorphan	66	None
		Aptiganel	94	NA
		Magnesium	86	1500
		Remacemide	29	NA
	Competitive			
	antagonist of glutamate activation site	Selfotel	141	NA
	antagonist of the glycine recognition site	Gavestinel	150	NA
	antagonist of the polyamine site	Eliprodil	300	900
postreceptor effects	Attenuator of nitric oxide	Lubeluzole	232	NA
	Ganglioside	Siagoside (GM1)	2063	None
Modulators of calcium influx[b]	Antagonists of voltage-gated calcium channels	Nimodipine	3518	1500
		Nicardipine	5	NA
		Flunarizine	459	NA
		Darodipine	19	NA
		Isradipine	240	None
		Lifarizine	147	None
Metabolic activators[c]		Protirelin	60	None
		Naftidrofuryl	1265	None
Antioedema agents[d]	Inhibitor of bradykinin release	NT-3 (neurotrophin)	220	NA
	Other	Corticosteroids	620	NA
		Mannitol	300	None
		Glycerol	1400	None
Inhibitors of leucocyte adhesion		Anti ICAM-1	NA	600
Free radical scavengers[e]	21-Aminosteroid	Tirilazad	1219	NA
Promoters of membrane repair[f]	Choline precursor	Citicoline	611	NA
Unknown	β-Adrenoceptor antagonist	Propranolol	302	None
	Opioid receptor antagonists	Naloxone	233	None
		Nalmefene	44	NA

a Other agents that possibly have effects at this site include lubeluzole and lifarizine.
b Other agents that possibly have this mechanism of action include magnesium, lubeluzole, eliprodil, remacemide, dextromethorphan, dextrorphan and propentofylline.
c Other agents that possibly have this mechanism of action include magnesium and glycerol.
d Propentofylline may also have this mechanism of action.
e Glycerol may also have this mechanism of action.
f Gangliosides may also have this mechanism of action.

EAA = excitatory amino acid; **GABA** = γ-aminobutyric acid; **ICAM-1** = intracellular adhesion molecule 1; **NA** = data not available; **NMDA** = *N*-methyl-D-aspartate; **RCT** = randomised controlled trials.

protection observed experimentally appears to be independent of the exact mechanism of action.

In this classification, we have separated agents modulating glutamatergic transmission from agents acting on voltage-gated calcium channels. This is because recent evidence suggests that inhibition of peri-infarct membrane depolarisations, with a resultant reduced neuronal energy expenditure, might actually be the key mechanism underlying the neuroprotective effects seen in experimental animals.[11]

The available evidence from phase II studies of the efficacy of agents that effect EAA systems is summarised in table II. The first agents to be tested in this class were antagonists of glutamatergic transmission at the NMDA receptor. Since then, a variety of agents acting at different sites on this receptor (fig. 1) have been developed.

4.1.1 Agents with Presynaptic Effects

Sodium Channel Modulators

Sibatrigine

The novel compound sibatrigine (619C89) is closely related to the anticonvulsant lamotrigine. It inhibits burst firing and presynaptic glutamate release from depolarised/anoxic neurons by an interaction with sodium channels.[52] This agent has been shown to be effective in a variety of experimental models of ischaemic stroke.[53]

Several phase II studies have been completed. Preliminary information on safety is available from these studies (see table II): the development of visual hallucinations was the limiting step in dose escalation in study 137-101. At a loading dose of 2.5 mg/kg and a maintenance dosage 1.25 mg/kg/8 hours for 3 days, 35% of patients developed visual hallucinations.[43] These were not usually distressing and did not require either discontinuation of the study drug or additional treatment.

Study 137-102 was a further phase II randomised controlled trial assessing a single loading dose of 2 mg/kg followed by discrete boluses of 1 mg/kg 8 hourly for 3 days. Although the data remain blinded, the major adverse event was visual hallucinations, which were seen in 9 of 68 patients (all treatment groups combined). Two of these patients required sedation for the hallucinations.

Preliminary pharmacokinetic studies suggest sibatrigine has an elimination half-life of about 24 hours in stroke patients (R. Mulrooney, personal communication).

Fos-Phenytoin

The anticonvulsant phenytoin blocks voltage-dependent sodium channels[52] and also has demonstrated efficacy in experimental models of ischaemic stroke.[54,55] Phase III trials of fos-phenytoin (a phenytoin prodrug) have recently commenced (see table I).

γ-Aminobutyric Acid (GABA) Receptor Agonists

Facilitators of inhibitory neuronal systems provide a more physiological method of inhibiting EAA neurotransmission.

γ-Aminobutyric acid (GABA), the major inhibitory neurotransmitter of the mammalian CNS, has not been formally evaluated in acute stroke. 432 patients in the subacute phase of stroke were randomised in a controlled trial comparing GABA with pyritinol (pyrithioxine) and placebo.[56]

Table II. Effects of agents modulating excitatory amino acid neurotransmission in patients with acute stroke reported in phase II studies

Agent	Trial design	No. patients enrolled (A/P ratio)	Dose range[a]	Results: adverse effects	Results: mortality	Results: functional outcomes (% with good outcome)	Ref.
Sibatrigine[b]	de	48 (3/1)	LD 0.5-2.5 mg/kg; MD 0.25-1.25 mg/kg/8h for 3 days	Visual hallucinations, nausea, vomiting, agitation, confusion, drowsiness	A 6/36 *vs* P 3/12	NR	43
Sibatrigine[c]	de	68 (2/1)	LD 2 mg/kg; MD 1 mg/kg/8h for 3 days	Visual hallucinations, nausea, vomiting, agitation, confusion, drowsiness	NR	NR	
Dextrorphan	de	66 (NR)	LD 60-150mg; MD 15-135 mg/h for 23h	Nystagmus, nausea, vomiting, somnolence, hallucinations, agitation, hypotension	NR	NR	44
Aptiganel	de	94 (3/1)	LD 10-30 μg/kg; MD 3-10 μg/kg/h for 4h	Headache, sedation, nausea, vomiting, confusion/disorientation, agitation, paraesthesias/dysaesthesias	NR	NR	45
Magnesium sulfate	pfd	26 (1/1)	LD 4 mmol over 10 min, then 40 mmol/8h; MD 10 mmol tid (po) for 5 days	None	A 2/13 *vs* P 3/13	Trend in favour of A	46
Magnesium sulfate	pfd	60 (1/1)	NR	None	A 6/30 *vs* P 7/30	A 70 *vs* P 60	47
Remacemide	de	29 (3/1)	200-600 mg/day for 3-6 days	Agitation, venous irritation	NR by treatment group	NR	48
Selfotel	de	32 (3/1)	1-2 mg/kg	Agitation, hallucinations, confusion, paranoia	12.5% in both groups	A 95 *vs* P 29	49
Selfotel	sb	109 (1/1)	1.5 mg/kg	Agitation, hallucinations, confusion, paranoia [seen more frequently with A than P (57 *vs* 18%)]	NR	A 88 *vs* P 65	50
Eliprodil		>300	3mg bid for 3 days; 10mg (po) for 11 days	NR	NR	NR	d
Lubeluzole[e]	pfd	232 (NR)	LD 7.5-15 mg/h; MD 10-20 mg/day for 5 days	NR	High dose A 35%, low dose A 6%, P 18%	High dose A 34, low dose A 44, P 36	51

a All drugs were administered intravenously, unless otherwise stated.

b Study 137-101.

c Study 137-102.

d Trial CVD 715 still in progress.

e Study LUB-INT-4.

A = active treatment; **bid** = twice daily; **de** = dose escalation; **LD** = loading dose; **MD** = maintenance dose; **NR** = not reported; **P** = placebo; **pfd** = pilot fixed dose; **po** = oral; **sb** = single bolus; **tid** = 3 times daily.

GABA was generally well tolerated, with only 5% of the treatment group reporting (mainly gastrointestinal) adverse events. No striking effects on death or clinical outcomes were observed.

Clomethiazole (chlormethiazole), a GABA receptor agonist, has demonstrated neuroprotective efficacy in a gerbil model of transient forebrain ischaemia.[57] This agent is being evaluated in a phase III controlled clinical trial in acute ischaemic stroke at a total dosage of 75 mg/kg administered over 24 hours (N.G. Wahlgren, unpublished observations).

Barbiturates

It has been suggested that barbiturate therapy may have neuroprotective activity by reducing the metabolic demands of ischaemic neurons. A small randomised controlled trial (n = 26) of low dose (anticonvulsant concentration) phenobarbital (phenobarbitone) did not show any significant effect on clinical outcomes.[58]

Adenosergic Agents

Adenosine receptor agonists and adenosine-potentiating agents have consistently demonstrated neuroprotective efficacy in experimental models of ischaemic stroke.[59] The potentially useful pharmacological actions of adenosine mimetics include:[59]

- presynaptic inhibition of glutamate release
- inhibition of voltage-gated calcium channels
- local cerebral vasodilation
- inhibition of both platelet and neutrophil function.

Propentofylline, which acts by inhibiting adenosine reuptake, at a dosage of 1200mg administered intravenously for 7 days showed a trend towards improved functional outcomes (nonsignificant improvement in median Barthel score in treatment-allocated groups) in a small randomised controlled trial of 30 patients with acute ischaemic stroke.[60]

4.1.2 N-Methyl-D-Aspartate (NMDA) Receptor Antagonists

Although there are at least four separate glutamate receptor sites (see section 3.2), randomised controlled trials in humans have only examined antagonists of the NMDA receptor subtype in patients with acute stroke; to our knowledge agents acting at the other sites remain untested clinically.

NMDA receptor antagonists can be broadly classified as either competitive or noncompetitive receptor antagonists. The noncompetitive antagonists interfere with ionic flux by binding to a receptor within the ion channel (see fig. 1). The competitive NMDA receptor antagonists act at one of three activation sites on the receptor complex. Experimentally, adverse behavioural effects have tended to occur at the same doses of noncompetitive antagonists as those required to achieve neuroprotection,[26] whereas the competitive antagonists given at dosages sufficient to be neuroprotective are less likely to cause adverse behavioural effects.[26]

Noncompetitive NMDA Receptor Antagonists

Dextromethorphan and Dextrorphan

Both dextromethorphan and its primary metabolite dextrorphan are noncompetitive NMDA receptor antagonists.

In a placebo-controlled, double-blind, crossover study, dextromethorphan was administered orally at a dosage of 60mg 4 times daily for 3 weeks to patients with a history of minor stroke or transient ischaemic attacks (TIA).[61] No clinical evidence of toxicity was seen in this study.

Dextrorphan is a more potent glutamate antagonist than dextromethorphan in both *in vitro* and *in vivo* models. In an ascending dose safety study (see table II), transient and reversible adverse events of dextrorphan included nystagmus, nausea, vomiting, somnolence, hallucinations and agitation.[44] These occurred in all patients treated with the active agent. Escalation of the loading dose was discontinued because 7 of 21 patients who received doses from 200 to 260 mg/kg had a rapid symptomatic, but reversible, falls in systolic blood pressure.

Preliminary pharmacokinetic studies revealed that dextrorphan has a plasma elimination half-life of 2 to 5 hours, a large volume of distribution (250 to 650L), and a high clearance (47 to 259 L/h). As the study was not designed to evaluate efficacy, neurological outcomes were not assessed beyond 48 hours and no data on longer term functional outcomes were reported.[44]

Aptiganel

94 patients have been randomised in a placebo-controlled, double-blind, dose-escalation safety study (see table II).[45] Overall, no clinically significant adverse haemodynamic effects were seen, although 2 actively treated patients required hypotensive therapy. Adverse events, occurring within 12 hours of treatment, were primarily of the CNS and gastrointestinal system, e.g. headache, sedation, nausea and vomiting, disorientation, and paraesthesias. Ten transient episodes of mild to moderate confusion and/or agitation occurred. These all resolved without sequelae. Functional outcomes were reported as being 'encouraging', but more data are awaited. Further trials were started in early 1996.

Magnesium

Intravenous magnesium therapy has been extensively tested in acute myocardial infarction and found to be well tolerated.[62,63] Magnesium has a variety of potentially useful pharmacological actions in acute stroke: in experimental animal models it has been demonstrated that magnesium ions may not only modulate NMDA receptor function, but also have activity as calcium antagonists, vasodilators and antiplatelet agents (see Limburg and Hijdra[64]).

In two small pilot studies (n = 60 and 26) [see table II],[46,47] magnesium sulfate was administered intravenously to patients with acute stroke. No adverse haemodynamic or other effects were seen, and the study treatment was generally well tolerated. There was a trend towards decreased mortality and improved functional outcome, as assessed by the Barthel index, in the treatment group in both studies (see table II). At least one large phase III controlled clinical trial in acute ischaemic stroke is planned.[65]

Remacemide

Remacemide produces a metabolite that has moderate affinity for the NMDA receptor and acts as a noncompetitive antagonist.[5]

Twenty-nine patients, presenting within 12 hours of onset of an acute middle cerebral artery territory stroke, were randomised in a dose-escalation study of this agent (see table II). The intravenous administration of remacemide was tolerated well in dosages up to 300mg twice daily. Data on clinical outcomes remain blinded to date.[48]

Competitive NMDA Receptor Antagonists

Selfotel

Thirty-two patients were enrolled in a double-blind ascending-dose study of selfotel (see table II).[49] Adverse effects (agitation, hallucinations, confusion, paranoia and delirium) occurred in all 6 patients treated with 6 mg/kg, and in 4 of 6 given 1.75 mg/kg. Similar, but milder, adverse effects were noted in 3 of 6 patients who received 1.5 mg/kg and 1 of 6 who received 1 mg/kg. These adverse events typically developed a mean of 1 to 3 hours after treatment, and the mean duration was approximately 24 hours. Treatment half-life ranged from 2 to 3.3 hours depending on dosage. Pooled mortality was 12.5% in both groups. There was a trend in favour of improved functional outcome on the Barthel index in the treatment group.

There has been a further report of a larger study of 109 patients treated with a single bolus intravenous injection of selfotel (1.5 mg/kg) or placebo within 6 hours of acute hemispheric stroke (see table II).[50] Similar adverse events were noted, with neurological adverse events (agitation, confusion, hallucinations) being seen more frequently in selfotel recipients (57%; 13% severe) than placebo recipients (18%; 0% severe). All adverse effects resolved within 72 hours. In this study, 88% of patients who received the drug were reported to have made a good recovery as assessed by the Barthel index compared with 65% in the placebo group.

Eliprodil

Eliprodil acts at the polyamine site of the NMDA receptor (see fig. 1). Trials of this agent began in April 1993, planning to recruit between 700 and 900 patients within 8 hours of stroke onset (see table II) [Cochrane Stroke Review Group, personal communication]. No further details are available at present.

Gavestinel

Phase II trials of this glycine site antagonist began in April 1995 (R. Mulrooney, personal communication). No published data are currently available.

4.1.3 Agents Effecting Postreceptor Mechanisms

Inhibitors of the Nitric Oxide System

Lubeluzole

Lubeluzole is the *S*-enantiomer of a novel benzothiazole compound. It has demonstrated neuroprotective efficacy in photochemically induced neocortical infarcts in rats,[66] and potently inhibits glutamate-activated elevations of cyclic guanosine monophosphate (cGMP) in animal models.[66] Therefore, it is speculated that the neuroprotectant activity of the drug may result from attenuation of glutamate-induced, NO-related neurotoxicity. Alternatively, its actions at the cell membrane (blockade of voltage-operated sodium and calcium channels[66]) may represent its primary mode of action.

In a recent phase II trial (LUB-INT-4),[51] 232 patients were treated either with placebo or an intravenous lubeluzole infusion over 1 hour, followed by a continuous 5-day infusion, at one of two dose levels. In patients who received the low-dose regimen, early case fatality was decreased (occurring in 6% of lubeluzole-treated *vs* 18% of placebo-treated patients) and improved functional outcomes were observed on the Barthel index (see table II). In contrast, the high-dose group had a higher early case fatality (35% lubeluzole-treated *vs* 18% placebo-treated) and worse functional outcomes.

These results appear rather extreme; the play of chance or the effects of imbalance in prognostic factors in the 3 treatment groups at randomisation may account for at least some of the observed differences, rather than any true benefits or hazards of the treatment itself. It seems unlikely that there are true qualitative differences between the low- and high-dose regimens (i.e. benefit with low-dose and harm with high-dose). Further studies of the lower dose regimen are underway (LUB-INT-5).

Siagoside (GM1)

Gangliosides are normal components of plasma membranes that are particularly abundant in the CNS. Their physiological role is believed to relate to regulating membrane-mediated cellular functions. There is *in vitro* evidence that they may limit EAA-mediated neurotoxicity, and this effect appears to occur solely by inhibition of the downstream consequences of EAA receptor stimulation.[67] Gangliosides may have additional useful functions in facilitating recovery post-stroke by the potentiation of endogenously occurring neuronotrophic factors.

There have been 12 randomised controlled trials of siagoside (GM1), which have included over 2000 patients with acute ischaemic stroke, and 9 of these trials have published data on the numbers of deaths in each treatment group.[68] A preliminary review of these data showed that siagoside had no effect on mortality (odds ratio 0.89; 95% confidence interval 0.71 to 1.11) [Cochrane Stroke Review Group, personal communication]. A systematic review of these trials is being prepared for the Stroke Module of the Cochrane Database of Systematic Reviews.[7]

Concerns that siagoside may be associated with the Guillain-Barré syndrome have led to the withdrawal of the product licence for this drug.

4.2 Modulators of Calcium Influx

Various agents that block predominantly L-type voltage-gated calcium channels have been tested in acute ischaemic stroke, including nimodipine,[69,70] nicardipine (Cochrane Stroke Review Group, personal communication), flunarizine,[64,71,72] darodipine (PY 108-068),[73] isradipine[74] and lifarizine (Cochrane Stroke Review Group, personal communication). In all, 23 randomised controlled trials have compared calcium antagonist therapy with control.

Nimodipine has now been tested in over 3500 patients, administered orally in most trials but intravenously in 4 trials.[75-78] Two systematic reviews have recently been published,[69,70] which included some of these trials. Both showed that nimodipine did not clearly reduce the risk of death or poor functional outcome. A subgroup analysis[70] suggested there might be some benefit if nimodipine therapy was started within 12 hours (although the same analysis suggested net harm if started more than 24 hours after stroke onset). Such subgroup analyses are particularly unreliable when the overall treatment effects are null and the apparent benefit may be purely the result of the play of chance.[79] A further trial of very early oral nimodipine (started within 6 hours of stroke onset) is being undertaken by primary health physicians in The Netherlands.[80]

Five other blockers of voltage-gated calcium channels have been examined in an additional 870 patients (see table I). We await a meta-analysis of all the trials of calcium antagonists, which is currently under preparation by the Cochrane Stroke Review Group.[7]

4.3 Metabolic Activators

4.3.1 Protirelin

Protirelin, or thyrotropin-releasing hormone, is a neuromodulator that may act on CNS cholinergic and monoaminergic neurotransmitter systems.[81] Although its potential mechanism of action is unclear, it has been evaluated in a single small nonblinded randomised controlled trial.[82] In this study, 60 patients were randomised within 15 days of acute stroke to either active treatment of protirelin 2 mg/ day for multiple 15-day cycles or placebo (1 : 1). Although the authors reported a statistically significant improvement in neurological score, this analysis took no account of those patients who died or who were lost to follow up. Reanalysis on a 'worst case scenario' revealed no clear difference between the treatment groups.

4.3.2 Naftidrofuryl

Naftidrofuryl has several potentially useful pharmacological actions, including vasodilation and the property of improving the efficiency of cerebral oxygen usage. There have been six randomised controlled trials[83-89] comparing the effect of the drug with control, involving approximately 1265 patients with acute ischaemic stroke. Overall, the available data do not provide reliable evidence of any clinical benefit.

A systematic review of these trials for the Cochrane database is planned (Cochrane Stroke Review Group, personal communication).

4.4 Antioedema Agents

Brain swelling, caused by cerebral oedema [cytotoxic (early and intracellular) or vasogenic (late and extracellular)], may contribute to the ischaemic neuronal damage that occurs in patients with acute stroke. Antioedema agents might have several useful pharmacological effects: (i) a reduction in cerebral oedema might limit ischaemic neuronal damage by an improvement in local blood flow; and (ii) it has also recently become clear that these agents have significant antioxidant activity that might limit free radical–mediated damage.

4.4.1 Corticosteroids and Mannitol

There have been 11 randomised controlled trials assessing the efficacy of corticosteroids in patients with predominantly acute ischaemic strokes. A provisional systematic review of 10 of these trials (n = 620), published only in abstract form, showed that treatment had no clear effect on mortality.[90] No information was available on the effect of treatment on functional outcome. Thus, the routine use of corticosteroids cannot be recommended.

A single small trial of mannitol in patients with acute stroke showed no benefit.[91]

4.4.2 Glycerol

Ten randomised controlled trials have compared glycerol with control in over 500 patients with acute stroke. Two systematic reviews[92,93] showed no overall effect on long term mortality, but one analysis did show a marginally significant reduction (42%) in the odds of death at 2 weeks.[92] A further large study of glycerol in 900 patients with acute ischaemic stroke is currently in progress [Trial Italiano sul Glicerolo Nell'Ictus (TIGI) Study].

4.4.3 NT-3 (Neurotrophin)

NT-3[94] (neurotrophin) is a nonprotein extract of cutaneous tissue from rabbits previously inoculated with the Vaccinia virus. It has recently been found to inhibit the release of bradykinin, an effect that leads to a reduction of oedema.[94]

A randomised controlled trial with NT-3[94] was recently performed in 220 patients admitted within 24 hours of acute ischaemic stroke. Patients were treated with an intravenous bolus of NT-3 (21.6mg) on admission followed by a continuous infusion (of 36mg) for 10 days. There was a trend in favour of the treatment group for mortality, functional outcome (assessed by the Toronto Stroke Score) and size of oedema zone assessed at 15 days. Unfortunately, interpretation of these results is hindered by the small number of patients, the exclusion of 76 of the randomised patients from the analysis, and the short duration of follow-up. Hyperglycaemia was the most frequent adverse effect in the treatment group, which may also have led to unblinding of outcome assessment in a large proportion of cases.

4.5 Inhibitors of Leucocyte Adhesion and Migration

Intracellular adhesion molecule 1 (ICAM-1) is a ligand on the endothelial cell surface that regulates leucocyte aggregation. It upregulates nonspecifically in the presence of inflammation. After brain ischaemia, ICAM-1 staining increases for 7 days. Antibodies to intracellular adhesion molecules, such as this, may block leucocyte-mediated cytotoxicity. In experimental models, blockade reduces infarct size in the middle cerebral artery occlusion model.[95]

A double-blind, randomised controlled trial,[96] aiming to recruit 600 patients, is currently being undertaken in patients with acute ischaemic stroke. Treatment will be started within 6 hours of stroke and continue for 5 days. The following adverse events are reported as 'common' in early phase clinical trials: nausea/vomiting, fever, headache and flushing.

4.6 Free Radical Scavengers and Antioxidants

Tirilazad is a 21-aminosteroid and a potent inhibitor of membrane lipid peroxidation and of activated oxygen species.[97] Results of a safety study in acute ischaemic stroke are available.[98] 111 patients were randomised to active drug or placebo (3 : 1). Treatment was given intravenously and started within 12 hours of stroke onset (median time 8.5 hours) and continued for 3 days. Three successive dosage tiers were tested: 0.6 mg/kg/day, 2.0 mg/ kg/day and 6.0 mg/kg/day. Tirilazad was well tolerated at all 3 doses, with no evidence of clinically significant adverse effects. An excess of deaths and worse functional outcomes were observed in the tirilazad-treated group, with the excess being greatest in the highest dosage tier. These results could have reflected an imbalance in the baseline characteristics of the treatment and control groups. Two larger randomised controlled trials of tirilazad 6 mg/kg/day recently stopped randomisation prematurely due to a lack of efficacy, after enrolment of only 1108 patients (planned sample size 2210).[99,100] Apart from an increase in local venous irritation, tirilazad was well tolerated in both studies. Further studies evaluating higher doses are planned.

4.7 Promoters of Neuronal Repair

Cholines are naturally occurring, endogenous compounds that are essential intermediates in the synthesis of phosphatidylcholine (PC), a major neuronal membrane lipid.

It is believed that administration of citicoline might have a beneficial therapeutic effect by increasing the synthesis of PC. Citicoline is reported as being effective in animal models of stroke.[101]

A double-blind, randomised controlled trial of citicoline (1 g/day intravenously for 14 days) enroling 272 patients was performed in Japan.[102] This study reported a low incidence of adverse events: headache (2.1%) and vertigo (1.2%). Provisional results of a trial of citicoline in 80 patients with acute ischaemic stroke have recently been reported. The treatment was tolerated well and associated with promising functional outcomes.[103] A larger double-blind, placebo-controlled randomised dose-ranging study is currently underway. This study recruited 259 patients within 24 hours of onset of ischaemic stroke, continuing treatment for 6 weeks.[104]

4.8 Agents with an Unknown Mechanism of Action

4.8.1 β-Adrenoceptor Antagonists

The utility of this class of agents in acute stroke was evaluated by the Beta Blockade in Acute Stroke (BEST) trial.[105] 302 patients with acute stroke were randomised within 48 hours of symptom onset. The trial was not large enough to provide reliable evidence on safety or efficacy.

4.8.2 Opioid Receptor Antagonists

Naloxone, an opioid receptor antagonist, has been evaluated in a number of small randomised controlled trials.[106-110] The drug has a variety of potentially useful pharmacological actions including:[111]

- antioxidant function
- modulation of transmembrane calcium flux
- stabilisation of lysosomal membranes
- inhibition of proteolysis
- attenuation of cerebral oedema
- attenuation of NMDA receptor-mediated neurotoxicity.

Five randomised controlled trials of naloxone have been completed in patients with acute stroke.[106-110] In these studies, 233 patients have been randomised to either naloxone or placebo. Unfortunately, information on long term functional outcomes and survival is available in only two of these studies, which together include 135 patients.[108,109] A preliminary meta-analysis of these data suggest that naloxone may have a favourable effect on mortality (odds ratio 0.33, 95% confidence interval 0.12 to 0.90). Although this result is statistically significant at conventional levels, it should be interpreted with caution as the numbers of patients involved are small and it takes no account of other clinically important outcomes.

Nalmefene is an opioid receptor antagonist with relative selectivity for κ receptors. It has recently been evaluated in a randomised controlled trial of 44 patients with ischaemic stroke, presenting within 6 hours of onset. 34 patients were randomised to nalmefene (0.05 mg/kg bolus and 0.01 mg/kg maintenance) and 10 to placebo for 24 hours. The treatment was tolerated well, with no significant adverse events reported. Favourable outcomes with respect to mortality and functioning at 3 months were observed in the treatment group.[112]

5. Promising Neuroprotective Strategies

The neuroprotective agents that have been test ed in humans so far may be considered as representing the visible tip of the 'neuroprotection iceberg.' Another review has identified several hundred other neuroprotective agents currently under experimental evaluation.[113]

5.1 Glycine Site Partial Agonists and Antagonists

The marked adverse neuropsychological and behavioural effects seen with NMDA receptor antagonists (see section 4.1.2) prompted the development of agents that modulate NMDA receptor function by other means (which, hopefully, would not lead to behavioural or cognitive adverse effects).

5.1.1 Amino Cyclopropane Carboxylic Acid

Amino cyclopropane carboxylic acid is a partial agonist of the glycine site on the NMDA receptor (see fig. 1), and has demonstrated neuroprotective action in animal models.[114] Phase

I safety trials have been performed at doses predicted to have a neuroprotective effect. In these studies, no drug related adverse events were reported.[114] Phase II studies of prophylactic treatment in coronary artery bypass graft surgery (a procedure often associated with minor stroke) are planned; to our knowledge, no studies in acute stroke are planned.

5.1.2 Licostinel

Preclinical studies of the glycine antagonist licostinel (ACEA 1021) have revealed a favourable safety profile.[115] There are no other publicly available data on this agent.

5.2 Modulators of Non-*N*-Methyl-D-Aspartate Receptors

The increasing body of neuroprotective data obtained experimentally with an AMPA antagonist, NNC 079202 (NBQX), in ischaemic stroke,[116] suggests that modulation of non-NMDA receptors may be a useful neuroprotective strategy in humans.

5.3 Endothelin Receptor Antagonists

Endothelin, a putative neurotransmitter and potent vasoconstrictor, is believed to play a role in the pathophysiology of neuronal ischaemia. Endothelin antagonists appear promising in experimental models and may be useful in a variety of cerebrovascular events.[117]

5.4 Nonpharmacological Treatment

Experimental studies have shown that relatively small reductions (2 to 3°C) in brain temperature may have cytoprotective effects.[118] The mechanism may relate, in part, to a reduction in cerebral metabolism with a resultant conservation of adenosine triphosphate. Alternatively, hypothermia may reduce the release of potentially neurotoxic EAAs. Despite the obvious promise of this approach we have been unable to find any randomised controlled trial of this treatment in stroke.

6. Conclusions

A bewilderingly large number of neuroprotective treatments are currently under development. A simple classification of these agents into broad groups on the basis of common potential mechanisms of action and adverse effects might be useful to clinicians interested in stroke; it would bring some order to a large mass of information, and facilitate comparisons of the many agents under development. The development of a robust (and pharmacologically rational) classification is however complicated by the incomplete understanding of the complex pathophysiological changes following stroke and because many agents have more than one mode of pharmacological action. At present, it is largely a matter of speculation for a given drug which of several mechanisms of action might account for any neuroprotective benefit. Given these limitations, our proposed classification should be viewed as an initial framework for clinicians that will require refinement as data from clinical trials and pharmacological studies accumulate.

The majority of the trials reviewed were phase II studies, performed under the auspices of the pharmaceutical industry. As a result of understandable commercial needs and confidentiality agreements, we generally did not have access to confidential data and were limited to reviewing published evidence. The review must have underestimated the number and classes of agents under development, and perhaps provided only a proportion of the available clinical evidence. A shifting of the 'ground rules' to allow a wider dissemination of information relating to trials in progress might be in the interests of both the pharmaceutical industry and the clinical trialists involved.

In spite of the fact that approximately 12 000 patients with acute ischaemic stroke have been randomised in more than 80 trials of 31 different agents, none of the agents reviewed have been clearly shown to be beneficial. This lack of evidence of efficacy does not indicate a lack of promise, but merely reflects the fact that the majority of the trials were small and did not have sufficient statistical power to reliably detect moderate degrees of efficacy.

Although these studies have not given clear information on efficacy, they have been useful in providing initial indications of tolerability. The adverse effect profiles of the agents reviewed appear to differ widely; ranging from the psychomimetic effects seen with nearly all the agents modulating EAA transmission to haemolysis with antioedema agents such as glycerol. Despite the fact that the short term behavioural effects may well limit the practicability of certain agents, more data on efficacy and longer term safety are needed before the utility of any novel treatment can be assessed. At present, there is insufficient evidence to exclude the possibility that these treatments cause serious long term adverse events or increased mortality. Thus, the routine use of any form of neuroprotective therapy in clinical practice cannot be justified at present.

Many of the neuroprotective agents reviewed are without effect on coagulation or platelet function. However, we have not identified any published reports of trials of neuroprotective therapy in patients with primary intracerebral haemorrhage. This might simply be a consequence of the traditional exclusion of this population of patients with acute stroke from trials of potentially hazardous treatments. Further randomised controlled trials, involving patients with both ischaemic *and* haemorrhagic stroke, are required to identify which of the currently available agents warrant testing in large trials with sufficient power to detect moderate, but worthwhile, differences in major clinical outcomes such as death or disability. At least one such 'mega trial' of neuroprotective therapy is now in the planning stage.

Acknowledgements

Dr Paul Dorman is supported by a UK Medical Research Council clinical training fellowship, Dr Carl Counsell is supported by a Wellcome Trust research training fellowship and Dr Peter Sandercock is supported by a grant from the UK Medical Research Council. We would like to acknowledge the help of Dr Robert Mulrooney, and also Ms Hazel Fraser and other members of the Cochrane Stroke Review Group in the preparation of this review.

References

1. Sandercock PAG, Celani MG, Ricci S. The likely public health impact in Europe of simple treatments for acute ischaemic stroke [abstract]. Cerebrovasc Dis 1992; 2: 236
2. Harris AI. Handicapped and impaired in Great Britain. London: HMSO, 1971
3. Sandercock PAG, Willems H. Medical treatment of acute ischaemic stroke. Lancet 1992; 339: 537-9
4. Counsell C, Sandercock PAG. The management of patients with acute ischaemic stroke. Curr Med Lit Geriatr 1995; 7 (4): 99-110
5. Muir KW, Lees KR. Clinical experience with excitatory amino acid antagonist drugs. Stroke 1995; 26: 503-13
6. Fisher M. Medical therapy for ischemic stroke. In: Fisher M, Bogousslavsky J, editors. Current reviews of cerebrovascular disease. Philadelphia: Current Medicine, 1993
7. The Cochrane Database of Systematic Reviews [database on disk and CD-ROM]. The Cochrane Collaboration; Issue 2. Oxford: Update and Software. London: BMJ Publishing Group, 1995
8. The OSTR Collaborative Group. The Ottawa Stroke Trials Registry Collaborative Group and the Development of the Ottawa Stroke Trials Registry (OSTR). Controlled Clin Trials 1994; 15: 503-11
9. Astrup J, Siesjo BK, Symon L. Thresholds in cerebral ischaemia: the ischaemic penumbra. Stroke 1981; 12: 723-5

10. Heiss W-D, Graf R. The ischaemic penumbra. Curr Opin Neurol 1994; 7: 11-9
11. Hossman K-A. Viability thresholds and the penumbra of focal ischemia. Ann Neurol 1994; 36: 557-65
12. Mies G, Iijima T, Hossman K-A. Correlation between peri-infarct DC shifts and ischaemic neuronal damage in rat. Neuroreport 1993; 4: 709-11
13. Shinohara M, Dollinger B, Brown G, et al. Cerebral glucose utilization: local changes during and after recovery from spreading cortical depression. Science 1979; 203: 188-90
14. Kocher M. Metabolic and haemodynamic activation of postischemic rat brain by cortical spreading depression. J Cereb Blood Flow Metab 1990; 10: 564-71
15. Choksey MS, Costa DC, Iannotti F, et al. 99TCm-HMPAO SPECT studies in traumatic intracerebral haematoma. J Neurol Neurosurg Psychiatry 1991; 54: 6-11
16. Nehls DG, Mendelow D, Graham DI, et al. Experimental intracerebral hemorrhage: progression of hemodynamic changes after production of a spontaneous mass lesion. Neurosurgery 1995; 23: 439-44
17. Choi DW. Excitotoxicity. In: Meldrum BS, editor. Excitatory amino acid antagonists. Oxford: Blackwell, 1991: 216-36
18. Rothman SM, Olney JW. Glutamate and the pathophysiology of hypoxic-ischaemic brain damage. Ann Neurol 1986; 19: 105-11
19. Baker AJ, Zornow MH, Scheller MS. Changes in extracellular concentrations of glutamate, aspartate, glycine, dopamine, serotonin and dopamine metabolites after transient global ischaemia in the rabbit brain. J Neurochem 1991; 57: 1370-9
20. Greenamyre JT, Porter RHP. Anatomy and physiology of glutamate in the CNS. Neurology 1994; 44 Suppl. 8: S7-S13
21. MacDermott AB, Mayer ML, Westbrook GL. NMDA-receptor activation increases cytoplasmic calcium concentration in cultured spinal cord neurones. Nature 1986; 321: 519-22
22. Rothman SM. Excitotoxins: possible mechanisms of action. Ann NY Acad Sci 1992; 648: 132-9
23. Butcher SP, Bullock R, Graham DI, et al. Correlation between amino acid release and neuropathological outcome in rat brain following middle cerebral artery occlusion. Stroke 1990; 21: 1727-33
24. Benveniste H, Drejer J, Schousboe A, et al. Elevation of extracellular concentrations of glutamate and aspartate in rat hippocampus during transient cerebral ischaemia monitored by intracerebral microdialysis. J Neurochem 1984; 43: 1369-74
25. Olney JW. Neurotoxicity of excitatory amino acids. In: McGeer EG, et al., editors. Kainic acid as a tool in neurobiology. New York: Raven Press, 1978: 37-70
26. McCulloch J. Excitatory amino acid antagonists and their potential for the treatment of ischaemic brain damage in man. Br J Clin Pharmacol 1992; 34: 106-14
27. Albers GW, Goldberg MP, Choi DW. Do NMDA antagonists prevent neuronal injury? Yes. Arch Neurol 1992; 49: 418-20
28. Choi DW. Nitric oxide: foe or friend to the injured brain? Proc Natl Acad Sci USA 1993; 90: 9741-3
29. Faraci FM, Brian JE. Nitric oxide and the cerebral circulation. Stroke 1994; 25: 692-703
30. Harris RJ, Symon L. Extracellular pH, potassium, and calcium activities in progressive ischaemia of rat cortex. J Cereb Blood Flow Metab 1984; 4: 178-86
31. Hossman K-A, Schuier FJ. Experimental brain infarcts in cats. I. Pathophysiological observations. Stroke 1980; 11: 583-92
32. Lipton SA, Rosenberg PA. Excitatory amino acids as a final common pathway for neurologic disorders. N Engl J Med 1994; 330: 613-22
33. Siesjo BK. Pathophysiology and treatment of focal cerebral ischaemia. Part II. Mechanisms of damage and treatment. J Neurosurg 1992; 77: 337-54
34. Belch JJF. Free radicals and their scavenging in stroke. Scot Med J 1992; 37 (3): 67-8
35. Kogure K, Kato H. Altered gene expression in cerebral ischaemia. Stroke 1993; 24: 2121-7
36. Harlan JM. Neutrophil mediated vascular injury. Acta Med Scand Suppl. 1985; 715: 123-9
37. Wiebers DO, Adams HP, Whisnant JP. Animal models of stroke: are they relevant to human disease? Stroke 1990; 21: 1-3
38. Wise RJS, Bernardi S, Frackowiak RSJ, et al. Serial observations on the pathophysiology of acute stroke. The transition from ischaemia to infarction as reflected in regional oxygen extraction. Brain 1983; 106: 197-222
39. Heiss WD, Huber M, Fink GR, et al. Progressive derangement of periinfarct viable tissue in ischemic stroke. J Cereb Blood Flow Metab 1992; 12: 193-203
40. Baron JC. Ischemic stroke studied by ^{15}O-labelled compounds: misery perfusion and luxury perfusion. In: Heiss WD, et al., editors. Clinical efficacy of positron emission tomography. Boston/Dortrecht: Martinus Nijhoff Publishing, 1987: 15-23
41. Heiss WD, Fink GR, Huber M, et al. Positron emission tomography imaging and the therapeutic window. Stroke 1993; 24 Suppl.: I-50-3
42. Warach S, Benfield A, Edelman RR. Prolonged evolution of lesion volume in human stroke determined by diffusion-weighted MRI [abstract]. Neurology 1995; 45 Suppl. 4: 287
43. Muir KW, Lees KR, Hamilton SJC, et al.. A randomised, double-blind, placebo-controlled ascending dose tolerance study of 619C89 in acute stroke [abstract]. Second International Conference on Neuroprotective Therapy: 1994 Jul 31-Aug 3; New York
44. Albers GW, Atkinson R, Kelley R, et al. on behalf of the Dextrorphan Study Group. Safety, tolerability, and pharmacokinetics of the N-methyl-D-aspartate antagonist dextrorphan in patients with acute stroke [abstract]. Stroke 1995; 26: 254-8
45. Fisher M, CNS 1102-003 Investigators. Cerestat (CNS 1102) a non-competitive NMDA antagonist, in ischemic stroke patients: dose-escalating safety study [abstract]. Cerebrovasc Dis 1994; 4: 245

46. Strand T, Wester PO, CVD Group. A double blind randomized pilot trial of magnesium therapy in acute cerebral infarction [abstract]. 7th Nordic Meeting on Cerebrovascular Disease; 1993 Aug 14-17; Jyräskylä, Finland, 1: 37
47. Muir KW, Lees KR. A randomized, double-blind, placebo-controlled pilot trial of intravenous magnesium sulfate in acute stroke. Stroke 1995; 26: 1183-8
48. Muir KW, Lees KR. Initial experience with remacemide hydrochloride in patients with acute ischaemic stroke [abstract]. Proceedings of the Second International Conference of Neuroprotective Agents; 1994 Jul 31-Aug 3; Lake George (NY)
49. Grotta J, CGS19755 Study Group. Safety and tolerability of the glutamate antagonist CGS19755 in acute stroke patients [abstract]. Stroke 1994; 25 (1): 255
50. Clark WM, Coull BM. Randomised trial of CGS19755, a glutamate antagonist, in acute ischaemic stroke treatment [abstract]. Neurology 1994; 44 Suppl. 2: A270
51. Diener HC, Hacke W, Hennerici M, et al. The effects of lubeluzole in the acute treatment of ischemic stroke: results of a Phase-2 trial [abstract]. Stroke 1995; 26: 185
52. Taylor CP, Meldrum BS. Na^+ channels as targets for neuroprotective drugs. Trends Pharmacol Sci 1995; 16: 309-16
53. Leach MJ, Swan JH, Eisenthal D, et al. BW 619C89, a glutamate release inhibitor, protects against focal cerebral ischaemic damage. Stroke 1993; 24: 1063-7
54. Boxer PA, Cordon JJ, Mann ME, et al. Comparison of phenytoin with non competitive NMDA antagonists in a model of focal brain ischemia in rat. Stroke 1990; 21 Suppl. III: 47-51
55. Rataud J, Debarnot F, Mary V, et al. Comparative study of voltage-sensitive sodium channel blockers in focal ischaemia and electric convulsions in rodents. Neurosci Lett 1994; 172: 19-23
56. Otomo E, Araki G, Mori A, et al. Clinical evaluation of GABA in the treatment of cerebrovascular disorders. Multi-center double blind study in comparison with pyrithioxine and placebo. Arzneimittelforschung 1981; 9: 1511-23
57. Cross AJ, Jones JA, Baldwin HA, et al. Neuroprotective activity of chlormethiazole following transient forebrain ischaemia in the gerbil. Br J Pharmacol 1991; 104: 406-11
58. Yatsu FM, Coull BM. Barbiturate therapy in stroke. In: Fisher M, editor. Medical therapy of acute stroke. New York, Basel: Marcel Dekker Inc., 1989: 109-15
59. Miller LP, Hsu C. Therapeutic potential for adenosine receptor activation in ischaemic brain injury. J Neurotrauma 1992; 9 Suppl. 2: S563-77
60. Huber M, Kittner B, Hojer C, et al. Effect of propentofylline on regional cerebral glucose metabolism in acute ischaemic stroke. J Cereb Blood Flow Metab 1993; 13: 526-30
61. Albers GW, Saenz RE, Moses JA, et al. Safety and tolerance of oral dextromethorphan in patients at risk for brain ischaemia. Stroke 1991; 22 (8): 1075-7
62. Woods KL, Fletcher S, Roffe C, et al. Intravenous magnesium sulphate in suspected acute myocardial infarction: the second Leicester Intravenous Magnesium Intervention Trial (LIMIT-2). Lancet 1994; 343: 1553-8
63. ISIS-4 Collaborative Group. ISIS-4: a randomised trial assessing early oral captopril, oral mononitrate, and intravenous magnesium sulphate in 58 050 patients with suspected acute myocardial infarction. Lancet 1995; 345: 669-85
64. Limburg M, Hijdra A. Flunarizine in acute ischemic stroke: a pilot study. In: Limburg M, editor. Stroke: aspects of diagnosis and management. Amsterdam: Rodopi, 1992: 81-4
65. Muir KW, Lees K. Intravenous magnesium efficacy in stroke (IMAGES) trial. Annual Meeting of the British Stroke Research Group: 1995 Jan; Leeds
66. De Ryck M. Lubeluzole: preclinical neuroprotective properties in relation to acute treatment of ischemic stroke. Recent advances in the understanding and therapy of ischaemic stroke: 1994 Nov 30-Dec 1; Philadelphia
67. Vaccarino F, Guidotti A, Costa E. Ganglioside inhibition of glutamate-mediated protein kinase C translocation in primary cultures of cerebellar neurons. Proc Natl Acad Sci USA 1987; 84: 8707-11
68. Argentino C, Sacchetti ML, Toni D, et al. GM1 ganglioside therapy in acute ischemic stroke. Italian Acute Stroke Study – Hemodilution + Drug. Stroke 1989; 20: 1143-9
69. Di Mascio R, Marchioli R, Tognoni G. From pharmacological promises to controlled clinical trials to meta-analysis and back: the case of nimodipine in cerebrovascular disorders. Clin Trial Meta-Analysis 1994; 29: 57-79
70. Mohr JP, Orgogozo JM, Hennerici M, et al. Meta-analysis of nimodipine trials in acute ischemic stroke. Cerebrovasc Dis 1994; 4: 197-203
71. Limburg M, Hijdra A. Flunarizine in acute ischemic stroke: a pilot study. Eur Neurol 1990; 30: 121-2
72. Prange H, Hartung J, Hertel G, et al. Treatment of acute stroke with flunarizine i.v. The German Flunarizine Study Group [abstract]. International Conference on Stroke: 1991 Geneva, Switzerland, 39
73. Oczkowski WJ, Hachinski VC, Bogousslavsky J, et al. A double-blind, randomized trial of PY108-068 in acute ischemic cerebral infarction. Stroke 1989; 20: 604-8
74. Azcona A, Lataste X. Isradipine in patients with acute ischaemic cerebral infarction: an overview of ASCLEPIOS programme. Drugs 1990; 40 Suppl. 2: 52-7
75. Bridgers SL, Koch G, Munera C, et al. Intravenous nimodipine in acute stroke: interim analysis of randomized trials [abstract]. Stroke 1991; 22: 153
76. Wahlgren NG, MacMahon DG, de Keyser J, et al. and the INWEST Study Group. Intravenous Nimodipine West European Stroke Trial (INWEST) of nimodipine in the treatment of acute ischaemic stroke. Cerebrovasc Dis 1994; 4: 204-10
77. Norris JW, LeBrun LH, Anderson BA, Canwin Study Group. Intravenous nimodipine in acute ischaemic stroke. Cerebrovasc Dis 1994; 4: 194-6
78. Heiss WD, Holthoff V, Pawlik G, et al. Effect of nimodipine on regional cerebral glucose metabolism in patients with acute ischemic stroke as measured by positron emmision tomography. J Cereb Blood Flow Metab 1990; 10: 127-32

79. Counsell CE, Clarke MJ, Slattery J, et al. The miracle of DICE therapy for acute stroke: fact or fictional product of subgroup analysis? BMJ 1994; 309: 1677-81
80. Limburg M, Horn J, Vermenten M. Very early nimodipine use in stroke (VENUS). Stoke 1996; 27: 361
81. Sharif NA. Diverse role of thyrotrophin-releasing hormone in brain, pituitary and spinal function. Trends Pharmacol Sci 1985; 6: 119-22
82. Montanari G, Fraioli P, Montemurro L, et al. Comparative study of protirelin tartrate and standard therapy in the treatment of stroke patients. Curr Therap Res 1994; 55: 1211-22
83. Admani AK. New approach to treatment of recent stroke. BMJ 1978; 2: 1678-9
84. Gray CS, French JM, Venables GS, et al. A randomized double-blind controlled trial of naftidrofuryl in acute stroke. Age Ageing 1990; 19: 356-63
85. Steiner TJ, Clifford Rose F. Randomized double-blind placebo-controlled clinical trial of naftidrofuryl in hemiparetic CT-proven acute cerebral hemisphere infarction. In: Clifford Rose F, editor. Stroke: epidemiological, therapeutic and socio-economic aspects. Royal Society of Medicine Services International Congress and Symposium Series No.99. London: Royal Society of Medicine Services Limited, 1986: 85-98
86. Steiner TJ. Praxilene in stroke treatment in Northern Europe (PRISTINE) [abstract]. Stroke 1994; 25: 544
87. Ohtomo E, Nakajima K, Araki G, et al. Clinical evaluation of LS-121 injection in the treatment of cerebral infarction and cerebral haemorrhage in acute and subacute stages – multi center double-blind study with placebo as the control drug. Clin Eval 1987; 15: 107-42
88. Steiner TJ, MacWalter R, Sanders E for the PRISTINE Group. Naftidrofuryl promote earlier recovery from acute cerebral infarction: principal results of the PRISTINE study [abstract]. Eur J Neurology 1995; 2: 122-3
89. Orgogozo JM, Lehert P, Mosnier M. Double-blind study of naftidrofuryl on secondary outcome after MCA infarction [abstract]. Cerebrovasc Dis 1995; 5: 235
90. Qizilbash N, Murphy M. Meta-analysis of trials of corticosteroids in acute stroke [abstract]. Age Ageing 1993; 22 Suppl. 2: 4
91. Santambrogio S, Martinotti R, Sardella F, et al. Is there a real treatment for stroke? Clinical and statistical comparison of different treatments in 300 patients. Stroke 1978; 9: 130-2
92. Rogvi-Hansen B, Boysen G. I.V. glycerol treatment in acute ischaemic stroke. In: Warlow C, Sandercock P, von Gign J. Stroke module of the Cochrane database of systematic reviews. London: BMJ Publishing, 1995
93. Qizilbash N, Murphy M. Meta-analysis of trials of glycerol in acute stroke [abstract)]. Age Ageing 1993; 22 Suppl. 2: 4
94. De Reuck J, Decoo D, Vanderdonckt P, et al. A double blind study of neurotropin in patients with acute ischaemic stroke. Acta Neurol Scand 1994; 89: 329-35
95. Zhang RL, Chopp M, Jiang M , et al. Anti-intracellular adhesion molecule-1 antibody reduces ischaemic cell damage after transient but not permanent middle cerebral artery occlusion in the Wistar rat. Stroke 1995; 26: 1438-43
96. Sherman DG, Polmar SH. Development of ICAM-1 for stroke: Enlimomab (a murine anti-ICAM-1 antibody) vs placebo in a double-blind randomised trial for ischaemic stroke treated within 6 hours of onset. Recent Advances in the Understanding and Therapy of Ischemic Stroke: 1994 Nov 30-Dec 1; Philadelphia
97. Smith DH, Gennarelli TA, McIntosh TK. The potential of 21-aminosteroids as neuroprotective therapies in CNS injury. CNS Drugs 1995; 3: 159-64
98. The STIPAS Investigators. Safety study of tirilazad mesylate in patients with acute ischemic stroke (STIPAS). Stroke 1994; 25: 418-23
99. Peters GR, Hwang L-J, Musch B, et al. Safety and efficacy of 6 mg/kg/day tirilazad mesylate in patients with acute ischaemic stroke (TESS study) [abstract]. Stroke 1996; 27 (1): 32
100. The RANTASS Investigators. Randomized trial of tirilazad in stroke (RANTASS) [abstract]. Stroke 1996; 27 (1): 32
101. Nilsson B. CDP-choline: a short review. In: Tognoni G, Garattini S, editors. Drug treatment and prevention in cerebrovascular disorders. Amsterdam: Elsevier, 1979: 273-7
102. Tazaki Y, Sakai F, Otomo E, et al. Treatment of acute cerebral infarction with a choline precursor in a multicenter double-blind placebo-controlled study. Stroke 1988; 19: 211-6
103. Guillen F, Buendia C, Herrera J. CDP-Choline in the treatment of acute ischaemic stroke [abstract]. J Neurol 1995; 242 Suppl. 2: S76
104. Sandage BW, Interneuron Pharmaceuticals. I. Citicoline: to promote stroke recovery [abstract]. Recent Advances in the Understanding and Therapy of Ischemic Stroke: 1994 Nov 3-Dec 1; Philadelphia
105. Barer DH, Cruickshank JM, Ebrahim SB, et al. Low dose beta blockade in acute stroke (‘BEST’ trial): an evaluation. BMJ 1988; 296: 737-41
106. Perraro F, Tosolini G, Pertoldi F, et al. Double-blind placebo-controlled trial of naloxone on motor deficits in acute cerebrovascular disease [letter]. Lancet 1984; 1: 915
107. Fallis RJ, Fisher M, Lobo RA. A double blind trial of naloxone in the treatment of acute stroke. Stroke 1984; 15: 627-9
108. Czlonkowska A, Mendel T, Baranska-Gieruszczak M. A double-blind controlled trial of naloxone in early treatment of acute stroke. Cerebrovasc Dis 1992; 2: 40-3
109. Federico F, Lucivero V, Lamberti P, et al. A double blind randomised pilot trial of naloxone in the treatment of acute ischemic stroke. Ital J Neurol Sci 1991; 12: 557-63
110. Czlonkowska A, Cyrta B. Effect of naloxone on acute stroke. Pharmacopsychiatry 1988; 21: 98-100
111. Faden AL. The role of opiate antagonists in the treatment of stroke. In: Weinstein PR, Faden AL, editors. Protection of the brain from ischaemia. Baltimore: Williams and Williams, 1990: 265-71
112. Clark WM, Coull B. Randomized trial of cervene, a kappa receptor selective opioid antagonist, in acute ischemic stroke [abstract]. Neurology 1995; 45 Suppl. 4: A241

113. Dick E, Jost BC, Wilp R. Stroke: focus on opportunity. St Louis: Medstrategy Inc., 1994
114. Maccecchini M-L. Partial agonism and neuroprotection [abstract]. Recent advances in the understanding and therapy of ischaemic stroke: 1994 Nov 30- Dec 1; Philadelphia
115. Whitehouse MG. Glycine antagonists – developmental issues for use as neuroprotectants [abstract]. Recent advances in the understanding and therapy of ischaemic stroke: 1994 Nov 30-Dec 1; Philadelphia
116. Lees GJ. Therapeutic potential of AMPA receptor ligands in neurological disorders. CNS Drugs 1996; 5: 51-74
117. Patel TR. Therapeutic potential of endothelin receptor antagonists in cerebrovascular disease. CNS Drugs 1996; 5: 293-310
118. Busto R, Dietrich W, Globus MY, et al. Small differences in intraischemic brain temperature critically determines the extent of neuronal injury. J Cereb Blood Flow Metab 1987; 7: 729-38

Correspondence : Dr *P.J. Dorman,* Neurosciences Trials Unit, Department of Clinical Neurosciences, University of Edinburgh, Western General Hospital, Crewe Road, Edinburgh EH4 2XU, Scotland.

Maximising Health Outcomes in Stroke

Ian Reeves[1,2] and *Peter Langhorne*[2]

1 Department of Medicine, Glasgow Royal Infirmary, Glasgow, Scotland
2 Academic Section of Geriatric Medicine, Glasgow Royal Infirmary, Glasgow, Scotland

Stroke is the third commonest cause of death and commonest cause of adult disability in most developed countries.[1] Measures to reduce the incidence of new or recurrent stroke or reduce the severity of stroke disease could have a major beneficial impact. This article reviews the evidence supporting interventions which aim to reduce this burden of stroke disease. Although stroke disease, in general, can include transient ischaemic attacks (TIA), cerebral infarction or intracerebral haemorrhage, it should be noted that some interventions (e.g. anticoagulation, carotid surgery) are directed specifically at cerebral infarction.

This article identifies relevant prevention strategies which can be applied in a clinical setting. The scope does not include details of how these strategies might be achieved. The risk factors for stroke disease are examined first and then relevant interventions are considered, i.e.:

- Primary prevention, which aims to reduce the incidence of stroke or TIA in individuals at risk.
- Secondary prevention, which aims to reduce recurrent stroke in those who have experienced a TIA or stroke.
- Tertiary prevention, which aims to reduce the impact of established stroke in terms of death, disability or handicap.

This article takes a 'population-based' view and considers the potential effectiveness of an intervention and the number of patients who may benefit. Detailed cost-benefit analysis is not attempted, however, the broad implications of interventions in terms of their resource use and acceptability are considered.

1. Methods

A MEDLINE search was used to identify relevant articles. To maximise the sensitivity and specificity of this search, we used search strategies developed by the American College of Physicians.[2] These strategies differ for each type of article (such as those about prognosis, harm, treatment or cost effectiveness) and make MEDLINE searching more comprehensive and relevant. This basic strategy was supplemented with searches of the Cochrane Library.[3] We have tried to use accepted levels of evidence for research studies,[4] focusing on those studies with a low risk of bias (particularly systematic reviews of randomised trials). In some cases this level of evidence was not available because of (i) limited randomised, controlled trial evidence; (ii) significant heterogeneity between randomised, controlled trials (which may render these techniques invalid); or (iii) the criteria not being applicable (i.e. observational risk factor studies). In these circumstances we have tried to focus on the best available evidence (such as methodologically sound case-control studies). The presentation of evidence has included information from both risk factor and intervention studies.

1.1 Risk Factor Studies

The relative importance of risk factors is presented, where possible, as 'the number needed to harm' (NNH). This expresses the risk of an adverse event (stroke or TIA) appearing over a period of time for a given number of people exposed to the risk factor.[4] In a hypothetical example: where a risk factor for stroke increases the risk (over 5 years) from 1 to 1.01%, this could be expressed as an approximate NNH of 1000 (over 5 years). This means that 1000 people would need to be exposed to the risk factor for 5 years to cause 1 adverse event (in this case a stroke). Explicitly expressing data this way can be more meaningful than quoting relative risks (e.g. odds ratios or relative risk reduction), which do not take into account the baseline or absolute risk of an event.

Calculating the NNH involves taking the relative risk or odds ratio plus an expected event rate or baseline risk (PEER) if they were not exposed to that risk. For example, two trials (A and B) may both have a relative risk of 2. Trial A has an event rate of 0.05%, trial B has one of 4.7%. The NNH for trial A is calculated as 2000, whereas trial B has an NNH of 21. Those who require further information are directed to published examples.[4]

$$\text{NNH} = \frac{\text{PEER (OR} - 1) + 1}{\text{PEER (OR} - 1) \times (1 - \text{PEER})}$$

where OR is the odds ratio and PEER is the patient expected event rate.

1.2 Intervention Studies

For studies which have looked at interventions, we have tried to make the results comparable by expressing the treatment effect as the 'number needed to treat' (NNT). This method of presenting data is more clinically meaningful than relative benefits, and explicitly demonstrates the magnitude of benefit that an intervention will confer on both populations and individuals as it takes into account the baseline risk of that population or individual.[5]

$$\text{NNT} = \frac{1}{b - c}$$

where b = absolute risk in control group and c = absolute risk in treated group.

For example, an intervention which reduces the annual risk of stroke from 10% (0.1) to 5% (0.05) would have an NNT of 1/(0.1 – 0.05), i.e. 20. This figure means that 20 people would need to be treated with the intervention over 1 year to prevent 1 adverse outcome.

Calculating the NNT from a study allows this to be used as a simple indicator of the magnitude of the effect of the intervention within a single study, meta-analysis or systematic review. It also facilitates the comparison of the treatment effects between studies. However, the results are only truly comparable if the baseline risk in the control groups is similar. For example, a small treatment effect in a high risk group will generate a larger (i.e. less impressive) NNT than a large effect in a low risk group. We have therefore shown the baseline risk used

Table I. Risk factors for stroke/transient ischaemic attacks

Risk factor	Study type	RR	No. needed to harm	Patient expected event rate (%)	Ref.
Hypertension	Meta-analysis; 9 studies; 10-year follow-up (mean)	OR 10-12[a]	77	0.2	6
Smoking	Meta-analysis; 32 studies (follow-up not stated)	RR 1.5	Insufficient raw data to calculate	Insufficient raw data to calculate	7
Diabetes mellitus	Cohort study; 7549 men (22-year follow-up)	RR 2.45	233	0.33	8
Atrial fibrillation	Framingham cohort	Low risk[b]	27	1.0	9
	5070 patients (34-year follow-up)	High risk[c]	6	5.7	
Cholesterol	Cohort study	RR 1.81[d]	30 866[e]	0.004	10
	350 997 patients (6-year follow-up)	RR 2.57[f]	10 617[e]	0.006	
Lifestyle	Cohort study of 832 men, 3 daily servings of fresh fruit or vegetables (20-year follow-up)	RR 0.78	43	11	11
Carotid artery stenosis	Cohort study (4.5-year follow-up)	Degree of stenosis[g]			12
		0 to 30%	355	1.8	
		90 to 99%	9	14.4	

a For a diastolic blood pressure of 105mm Hg compared with 75mm Hg.
b Low risk = <65 years old with no additional risk factors.
c High risk = >65 years old plus one additional risk factor (e.g. heart failure, hypertension).
d For a cholesterol level of 6.19-7.22 mmol/L.
e The number needed to harm is large because death is used rather than stroke incidence. Assuming a 10% death rate, the number needed to harm would be 10 times smaller for stroke incidence, i.e. 3086 and 1061 respectively.
f For a cholesterol level of >7.22 mmol/L.
g Unable to calculate OR or RR.
OR = odds ratio; **RR** = relative risk.

to calculate NNT, but have not adjusted the NNTs to a common baseline risk. Readers interested in learning how to calculate NNTs are referred elsewhere.[4]

2. Potential Risk Factors

The search strategy identified seven potential risk factors for stroke which have been subject to detailed study (large cohort studies or randomised trials). These are outlined in table I and include:

- Blood pressure: there is a large amount of robust evidence indicating that hypertension is an important risk factor for stroke.[6] The level of risk increases with the level of blood pressure. The figures shown in table I refer to the increased risk of suffering a stroke if an individual has a diastolic blood pressure of 105mm Hg compared with 75mm Hg. As hypertension is both common and carries significant risk of stroke, it is generally considered to be the major risk factor for cerebrovascular disease.
- Cigarette smoking: there are considerable observational data[7] indicating that smoking approximately doubles the risk of stroke. This, too, is highly prevalent in many populations and hence a major risk factor.
- Diabetes mellitus: cohort studies with prolonged follow-up have indicated an approximate doubling of stroke risk in individuals with diabetes mellitus.[8] Less information is available for diabetes than for many other risk factors.
- Atrial fibrillation: nonrheumatic atrial fibrillation carries a significantly increased risk of stroke which varies according to other patient characteristics. Data from the Framingham study[9] indicated that older individuals (>65 years) who are in atrial fibrillation and who have additional vascular disease (e.g. heart failure, hypertension) are at increased risk of suffering a stroke compared with those under 65 years with no additional risk factors.

Table II. Treatment of risk factors for stroke/transient ischaemic attacks (primary prevention)

Risk factor	Type of study	ARR	No. needed to treat (1/ARR)	Outcome	Patient expected event rate (%)	Ref.
Hypertension	Meta-analysis	Data not available	319 181	Stroke mortality Stroke morbidity	0.95 1.5	13
	RCT; 4736 patients; systolic BP 130 to 210mm Hg	8.2 to 5.2% (3%, 0.03)	33	Total incidence of stroke	8.2	14
	Meta-analysis of 6 trials	Raw data not in paper	43	Cerebrovascular, mortality and morbidity	Data not published	15
Smoking cessation	Cochrane systematic review; RCT	0.06[a]	16	Smoking cessation; not stroke incidence or mortality	NA[a] NA[a]	16
		6.0 to 1.2%[a] 4.8%, 0.048 23.3 to 7.5%[a] 15.8%, 0.158	21[b] 6[c]	Smoking cessation; not stroke incidence or mortality	NA[a]	17
Cholesterol	Meta-analysis of diet or drug therapy; 46 538 men in 13 trials	Not calculated[d]	Not calculated[d]	All strokes	0.95	18
	RCT; pravastatin as primary prevention	0.019 to 0.017%	430	Primary outcome was cardiovascular, but stroke events were also measured	0.019	19
Atrial fibrillation	Meta-analysis of 33 studies	1.4 to 1% (0.4%, 0.04) 5.7 to 1.7% (4%, 0.4)	250 low risk[e] 25 high risk[f]	All strokes All strokes	1 5.7	20
Asymptomatic carotid artery stenosis	RCT	6.2 to 4.0% (2.2%, 0.02)	45	Strokes and death at 2.7 years	6.2	21
Thrombosis	Meta-analysis of antiplatelet agents	High risk 2.9 to 2.1% Low risk 1.15 to 0.95%	125 500	Strokes (non-fatal)	2.9 0.95	22

a Study measured smoking cessation, not stroke outcome.

b For most severe definition of smoking cessation (urine testing) and a 'high intervention' strategy.

c For least severe definition of smoking cessation (self reporting) and a 'high intervention' strategy.

d As wide confidence intervals suggest no benefit.

e Low risk = <65 years old with no additional risk factors.

f High risk = >65 years old plus one additional risk factor (e.g. heart failure, hypertension).

ARR = absolute risk reduction; **BP** = blood pressure; **NA** = not applicable; **RCT** = randomised control trial.

Table III. Secondary prevention of stroke/transient ischaemic attacks

Risk factor	Study	Type of study	ARR	No. needed to treat (1/ARR)	Outcome measure	Ref.
Hypertension	HSCSG	RCT	19.2 to 15.9% (3.3%, 0.033)	30	No. of strokes	23
Cholesterol	4S study	RCT of simvastatin[a] in 4444 patients	4.3 to 2.7% (1.6%, 0.016)	62.5	No. of stroke events[b]	24
Atrial fibrillation	EAFT (warfarin)	RCT of 1007 patients[c]	12 to 4% (8%, 0.08)	12.5	No. of strokes	25
	EAFT [aspirin (acetylsalicylic acid)]		12.5 to 10.5% (2%, 0.02)	50		25
Thrombosis	Antiplatelet Trialists Collaboration	Systematic review[b]	22 to 18% (4%, 0.04)	25	No. of strokes	22
Carotid stenosis	NASCET 1991	RCT (stenosis 70 to 99%)	13.1 to 2.5% (10.6%, 0.106)	9.5	No. of ipsilateral strokes	26
	ECST 1996	RCT (stenosis 30 to 69%)	No benefit	NA	No. of ipsilateral strokes	27

a In myocardial infarction patients with hypercholesterolaemia.
b Primary outcome was cardiovascular disease although stroke events were also measured.
c Patients had suffered a transient ischaemic attack or minor stroke, given warfarin or aspirin depending on bleeding risk.
ARR = absolute risk reduction; **EAFT** = European Atrial Fibrillation Trial; **ECST** = European Carotid Surgery Trial; **HSCSG** = Hypertension Cooperative Study Group; **NA** = not applicable; **NASCET** = North American Symptomatic Carotid Endarterectomy Trial; **RCT** = randomised control trial.

These are important observations when it comes to selecting patients for prevention measures (see tables II and III).

- Cholesterol: although cholesterol is well established as a risk factor for ischaemic heart disease, its role in cerebrovascular disease has been more controversial. Recent large studies[10] have indicated that higher levels of serum cholesterol do confer an increased risk of stroke.
- Lifestyle: some evidence has emerged to indicate that aspects of lifestyle including diet (fresh fruit or vegetables) and exercise[11] may influence the risk of stroke. There is relatively little information available at present in comparison with other risk factors.
- Carotid artery stenosis: there is valid evidence to indicate that an asymptomatic carotid artery stenosis increases the risk of an ipsilateral cerebral infarction or TIA.[12] The level of risk increases with both the degree of stenosis[27] and whether symptoms have been present (i.e. an asymptomatic stenosis carries less risk of major stroke than a recently symptomatic stenosis).[12] This has implications when selecting prevention measures.

Taking into account the prevalence of individual risk factors and the risk which they confer, it would appear that hypertension, cigarette smoking, nonrheumatic atrial fibrillation, diabetes mellitus and aspects of lifestyle are the major risk factors currently identified. Carotid stenosis is important at an individual level but less so at a population level. The NNH information is useful for identifying high-risk populations but it should be recognised that within these populations there will be considerable variation in risk. Recent studies have shown how data on several cardiovascular risk factors may be combined to help stratify patients at risk of ischaemic heart disease.[28] Similar data would be very useful to estimate an individual's risk of cerebrovascular disease.

3. Primary Prevention

Primary prevention interventions target recognised risk factors with the aim of reducing the incidence of first stroke. As noted in section 2, there are several risk factors which can predict an increased risk of stroke. In table II, 6 primary prevention strategies are identified which address the risk factors outlined in table I and are supported by valid evidence from randomised trials (table II). The main primary prevention strategies identified were directed at:

- treatment of hypertension
- smoking cessation
- anticoagulation in atrial fibrillation
- cholesterol reduction
- diabetic control
- carotid artery stenosis.

There is unequivocal evidence that treatment of hypertension reduces the incidence of stroke. However, the benefit obtained from treating hypertension varies with the baseline risk of the population being treated. Thus, the initial hypertension trials showed only relatively small benefits, i.e. a large NNT to prevent 1 stroke.[13] However, later studies[14,15] which have focused on groups with a higher baseline risk (e.g. the elderly) have shown much more impressive findings.

Recent systematic reviews and randomised, controlled trials of strategies for smoking cessation[16,17] have demonstrated that effective programmes do exist. What is lacking is direct evidence that these changes reduce stroke incidence. However, we could infer that this is the case from observational studies[29] showing that the risk of stroke in individuals who stop smoking returns to that of nonsmokers after a 4-year period (and so the NNT for smoking cessation in preventing stroke is probably quite small).

Substantial evidence from randomised controlled trials, confirmed by systematic reviews of randomised trials,[19] indicates that anticoagulation is effective at reducing stroke in individuals with nonrheumatic atrial fibrillation.[20] Once again, the absolute benefit from anticoagulation varies with the baseline risk of the individuals treated. A recent pooled analysis[20] demonstrated that older individuals with other vascular disease (hypertension, diabetes) are at the greatest risk of stroke and so enjoy the greatest absolute benefit from anticoagulation with warfarin. Younger individuals (<65 years) with no risk factors obtained no substantial benefit.

The alternative to full anticoagulation with warfarin is antithrombotic therapy with aspirin, which is probably less effective but safer. Low dose aspirin is therefore recommended for low risk individuals and those with contraindications to warfarin.[20,22] One major limitation in all the atrial fibrillation trials is the high degree of selection of patients at recruitment. It is therefore difficult to be certain how safe and reliable anticoagulation is in the elderly population in general.

There is limited reliable information available at present regarding the role of cholesterol reduction in preventing stroke. A meta-analysis of diet and drug therapy trials[18] showed wide confidence intervals consistent with no benefit. However, a more recent study of pravastatin in men at high risk of having vascular disease[19] indicated a clear reduction of cardiovascular outcomes and a potential reduction in stroke. Further information should become available from ongoing cholesterol-lowering studies.

The role of carotid endarterectomy in primary prevention of stroke (i.e. for asymptomatic carotid artery stenosis) is currently controversial. A recent randomised trial[21] has shown that surgery is effective at reducing stroke incidence but the absolute benefit is relatively small. This small benefit has to be balanced against the risks of surgery and the substantial costs of screening and surgery. Any small rise in the perioperative risk (3% combined mortality and morbidity) could negate any benefit from the operation.

There are few studies available directly linking improved diabetic control with a reduced risk of stroke. However, there are other good reasons (such as prevention of nephropathy, retinopathy and neuropathy) to justify good diabetic control.

4. Secondary Prevention

Secondary prevention measures aim to reduce recurrent stroke in those who have suffered a TIA or stroke. We identified five main secondary prevention measures which have been calculated by randomised trials or higher levels of evidence such as meta-analyses (table III). The prevention measures identified were as follows:

- blood pressure reduction
- cholesterol reduction
- anticoagulation in atrial fibrillation
- low dose aspirin
- endarterectomy for carotid stenosis.

There is little direct evidence regarding blood pressure reduction in individuals who have already suffered stroke or TIA. The available evidence suggests that this may be an effective strategy[23] but at least 2 large randomised trials should provide more information in the near future.

There is limited direct evidence about the role of cholesterol reduction in individuals who have previously suffered a stroke or TIA. There is indirect evidence from a large randomised trial[24] of cholesterol reduction for ischaemic heart disease which indicates a potential role for cholesterol reduction. More information should become available from ongoing randomised trials.

A large randomised trial[25] has shown unequivocal benefit of anticoagulation with warfarin for the secondary prevention of stroke. For those unable to tolerate warfarin there is some evidence to suggest that aspirin is an (less effective) alternative. The main clinical dilemma with individual patients is balancing the clear benefits of warfarin with the potential risks of anticoagulation.

There is overwhelming evidence to support the routine use of low dose aspirin (75 to 300 mg/day) in the secondary prevention of vascular disease (ischaemic heart disease, peripheral vascular disease, stroke and TIAs).[22] This is an important finding in population terms as aspirin use is acceptable, safe and widely applicable. Aspirin should be routinely provided as secondary prevention to individuals who have suffered a previous stroke or TIA, unless there are contraindications such as gastrointestinal bleeding or aspirin intolerance.

Two large randomised trials[19,26] have demonstrated the benefit of carotid surgery for symptomatic, severe (70 to 99%) carotid stenosis. At lower levels of stenosis there appears to be no overall benefit from surgery.[27] With an NNT figure of 10, carotid surgery for severe symptomatic carotid stenosis is highly effective at an individual patient level. However, in view of

Table IV. Summary of interventions to reduce the burden of stroke. Approximate values are given for key variables (based on tables I to III and Warlow et al.[32])

Intervention	No. who could benefit[a]	Absolute benefit in those at risk[b]	Potential hazard[c]	Potential cost[d]	Conclusion[e]
Primary Prevention					
Blood pressure reduction	Large	Medium	Low	Low-Medium	Recommended (both populations and high risk individuals)
Smoking cessation	?Large	?Medium	Low	Low-Medium	Recommended
Cholesterol reduction	Large	?Small	?Low	?Medium	Await RCT information (treat concomitant heart disease risk)
Anticoagulation in AF	Medium	Medium	?Medium	Medium	Select patients at high risk of stroke
Aspirin (acetylsalicylic acid) in AF	Medium	Medium	Low	Low	Routine if anticoagulation contraindicated
Asymptomatic carotid stenosis	Medium	Medium	?Medium	High	Routine screening and intervention *not* justified
Secondary prevention					
Aspirin (in sinus rhythm)	Medium	Medium	Low	Low	Routine use recommended
Aspirin (in AF)	Medium	?Medium	Low	Low	Routine (if anticoagulation contraindicated)
Anticoagulation in AF	Medium	Large	High	Medium	Select patients at low risk of complications
Symptomatic severe carotid artery stenosis	Small	Large	Medium	High	Selected patients only
Tertiary prevention					
Organised inpatient (stroke unit) care	Medium	Medium	Low	High (but similar to conventional care)	Routine use recommended

a Proportion of population who may benefit – small <1%; medium 1-10%; large >10%.
b Number needed to treat (NNT) to prevent 1 adverse outcome in 1 year – small (NNT >100); medium (NNT = 20-100); large (NNT <20).
c Subjective view based on potential harm of intervention if applied widely.
d Subjective view of resource implication of intervention.
e Subjective conclusion based on a, b, c and d.
AF = atrial fibrillation; **RCT** = randomised controlled trial; **?** = uncertain.

the relatively low prevalence of the risk factor, plus the potential risk and high cost of the operation, carotid surgery is unlikely to influence stroke incidence at a population level.

When considering secondary prevention interventions it is clear that there is a value in identifying individuals at highest risk of suffering a recurrent stroke as they stand to gain the greatest benefit from the intervention strategies. This principle applies to selecting those at high risk of stroke in the presence of atrial fibrillation, and those at high risk of stroke in the presence of carotid artery stenosis. For this reason, secondary prevention measures will frequently have to be tailored to the individual patient (table IV).

5. Tertiary Prevention

The aim of tertiary prevention is to reduce the impact of stroke by reducing disability and handicap. We have identified three possible options for tertiary prevention:

- acute drug therapies
- specific rehabilitation therapies
- organisational interventions

Despite a large amount of research activity there are as yet no proven routine therapies for acute stroke or drug therapies to improve recovery after stroke. There has been one encouraging trial of tPA in a very selected patient group[30] but we lack evidence to support widespread use. More information should be available in the near future regarding aspirin and heparin.

A large number of nonmedical and nonsurgical rehabilitation therapies are routinely used during stroke rehabilitation. Many are established routine practices although it is not possible to identify supporting evidence from the randomised control trials. We cannot at present comment on the population impact of these interventions.

The bulk of evidence regarding the effectiveness of different systems of delivering care for stroke patients concerns organised inpatient (stroke unit) care. To date, 19 randomised trials have compared organised stroke unit care with conventional care in a general ward.[31] Within trials which studied a relatively unselected population of stroke patients admitted to hospital (probably representing approximately 50 to 75% of all stroke patients) the NNT for prevention of death over 1 year was 22, prevention of death or disability was 16, prevention of death or need for institutional care was 14.[31] Cost-effectiveness studies are not available but most stroke units studied consumed approximately the same amount of resources as the general ward settings and so appear to be achieving better outcomes for little or no increased cost.

There has been recent interest in some countries in alternatives to hospital care (hospital-at-home, early supported discharge schemes) and although many are the subject of randomised trials, there is currently no information available on their effectiveness.

6. Conclusions

In this article we attempt to summarise the best identifiable evidence regarding recognised risk factors for cerebrovascular disease and interventions to reduce the incidence of first stroke, recurrent stroke or the complications of stroke. How then can we distil this information into simple conclusions regarding the current role of different interventions?

In making such decisions we have to consider the level of evidence supporting an intervention, the number of patients at risk within a population who are likely to gain benefit, the absolute benefit gained by those at risk, and any potential hazards or costs of the intervention. In the absence of detailed information to support all aspects of this decision-making process we have attempted to summarise the available information (in table IV) incorporating some value judgements about the relative benefit, hazards and costs of different interventions.

Blood pressure reduction would appear to have a major role in stroke prevention. The greatest public health impact would probably be achieved (e.g. by reducing salt in processed food) through a small reduction (e.g. 3mm Hg) in the average blood pressure in the population.[32] While drug treatment of individuals with high blood pressure is clearly important at an individual level, it is less likely to greatly influence the incidence of stroke. Smoking cessation programmes are probably also indicated, although we lack direct evidence to link smoking cessation with stroke reduction. Similarly, anticoagulation for high risk individuals in atrial fibrillation appears to be justified, with aspirin offered to those at lower risk. At present we lack evidence for cholesterol reduction as primary prevention of stroke, although it will frequently be indicated in an individual patient to reduce a concomitant risk of ischaemic heart disease. In view of the relatively low prevalence of carotid stenosis, the high cost of screening and the potential hazard of operation we do not believe there is currently a strong case for routine screening for asymptomatic carotid stenosis.

Secondary prevention measures should include the routine use of aspirin for all patients in sinus rhythm who have suffered a previous stroke or TIA (or other symptomatic vascular disease). Warfarin should be considered for all those in atrial fibrillation and aspirin given to those who have contraindications to warfarin. Carotid artery surgery should be reserved for those with a recently (in the last 6 months) symptomatic, severe (>70%) carotid artery stenosis. We lack direct evidence to support blood pressure reduction as a secondary prevention measure but further information should be forthcoming in the near future.

The only tertiary prevention intervention so far identified which could have an impact at a population level is the provision of organised multidisciplinary stroke unit care which appears to reduce the risk of death and disability after stroke. The costs of this intervention are probably comparable with the conventional care provided.

It is clear that we have evidence to support a number of stroke prevention strategies. The challenge now is to ensure that these strategies can be applied in an effective and efficient manner to reduce the burden of stroke.

References

1. Warlow C. Disorders of the cerebral circulation. In: Walton J, editor. Brains diseases of the nervous system. 10th ed. Oxford: Oxford University Press, 1993
2. How to harness Medline for prognosis problems [editorial]. ACP J Club 1995 Jul-Aug; 123: A12
3. Wimlow C, van Gijn J, Sandercock P, editors. Stroke module of the Cochrane Database of Systematic Reviews. Available in the Cochrane library. The Cochrane Collaboration, issue 1. Oxford: Update Software, 1997
4. Sackett D, Rosenberg W, Richardson S, et al. How to practise and teach evidence based medicine. Edinburgh: Churchill Livingstone, 1996
5. Sackett DL, Haynes RB, Guyatt GH, et al. Clinical epidemiology: a basic science for clinical medicine. 2nd ed. Boston (MA): Little, Brown and Co., 1991
6. McMahon S, Peto R, Cutler J, et al. Blood pressure, stroke, and coronary heart disease. Lancet 1990; 335: 765-74
7. Shinton R, Beevers G. Meta-analysis of relation between cigarette smoking and stroke. BMJ 1989; 298: 789-94
8. Burchfiel CM, Curb J, Rodriguez B. Glucose intolerance and 22-year stroke incidence. Stroke 1994: 25: 951-7
9. Wolf P, Abbot RD, Kannet WB, et al. Atrial fibrillation as an independent risk factor for stroke: the Framingham Study. Stroke 1991; 22: 983-8
10. Iso H, Jacobs D, Wentworth D, et al. Serum cholesterol levels and 6-year mortality from stroke in 350,977 men screened for the MRFIT. N Engl J Med 1989; 320: 904-10
11. Gilman M, Cupples A, Gasgon D, et al. Protective effect of fruits and vegetables on development of stroke in men. JAMA 1995; 73: 1113-7
12. European Carotid Surgery Trialists Collaborative Group. Risk of stroke in the distribution of an asymptomatic carotid artery. Lancet 1995; 345: 209-12
13. Insua J, Sachs H, Laut TC, et al. Drug treatment of hypertension in the elderly: a meta-analysis. Ann Intern Med 1994; 121: 355-62
14. Systolic Hypertension in Elderly Persons Co-operative Research Group (SHEP). Prevention of stroke by antihypertensive drug treatment in older persons with isolated systolic hypertension. JAMA 1991; 265: 3255-64
15. Mulrow C, Cornel J, Herrerac CR, et al. Hypertension in the elderly. JAMA 1994; 272: 1932-8
16. Silagy C, Ketteridge S. The effectiveness of physician advice to aid smoking cessation. The Cochrane library. The Cochrane Collaboration, issue 1. Oxford: Update Software, 1997
17. Weisfeldt J, Holloway J. Treatment for cigarette smoking in a Department of Veterans Affairs out-patient clinic. Arch Intern Med 1991; 151: 973-7
18. Atkins D, Psaty BM, Koepsell TD, et al. Cholesterol reduction and the risk of stroke in men: a meta-analysis of randomised controlled trials. Ann Intern Med 1993; 119: 136-45
19. Shepherd J, Cobbe SM, Ford I, et al. West of Scotland Coronary Prevention Study. N Engl J Med 1995: 333 (20): 1301-7
20. Matchar DB, McCrory DC, Barnett HJ, et al. Medical treatment for stroke prevention. Ann Intern Med 1994: 121 (1): 41-53
21. Asymptomatic Carotid Artery Stenosis (ACAS) study. Endarterectomy for asymptomatic carotid artery stenosis. JAMA 1995; 273: 1421-8
22. Antiplatelet Trialists Collaboration. Collaborative overview of randomised trials of antiplatelet therapy. BMJ 1994; 308: 81-106

23. Hypertension/Co-operative Study Group. Effective antihypertensive treatment on stroke recurrence. JAMA 1974; 229: 409-18
24. Scandinavian Simvastatin Survival Study Group (4S) Study. Randomised trial of cholesterol lowering in 4444 patients with coronary heart disease. Lancet 1994; 344: 1383-9
25. European Atrial Fibrillation Trial (EAFT) Study Group. Secondary prevention in non-rheumatic atrial fibrillation after transient ischemic attack or minor stroke. Lancet 1993; 342: 1255-62
26. North American Symptomatic Carotid Endarterectomy Trial (NASCET). Beneficial effect of carotid endarterectomy in symptomatic patients with high grade carotid stenosis. N Engl J Med 1991; 325: 445-53
27. Medical Research Council (MRC) European Carotid Surgery Trial. Interim results for symptomatic patients with severe (70-99%) and mild (0-30%) carotid stenosis: European Carotid Surgery Trialists Collaborative Group. Lancet 1991; 337: 1235-43
28. Jackson R. Available at the Centre for Evidence Based Medicine, http://www.cebm.jr2.0x.ac.uk
29. Kawachi I, Graham A, Colditz MD, et al. Smoking cessation and decreased risk of stroke in women. JAMA 1993; 269: 232-6
30. National Institute of Neurological Disorders and Stroke tPA Stroke Study Group. Tissue plasminogen activator for acute ischaemic stroke. N Engl J Med 1995; 333: 1581-7
31. Stroke Unit Trialists Collaboration. A collaborative systematic review of organised in-patient (stroke unit) care after stroke. BMJ. In press
32. Warlow CP, Dennis MS, van Gijn J, et al. Stroke: a practical guide to management. Edinburg: Blackwell Science, 1996

Correspondence: Dr *P. Langhorne,* Academic Section of Geriatric Medicine, 3rd Floor Centre Block, Glasgow Royal Infirmary, G4 0SF, Scotland.
E-mail: pl11m@clinmed.gla.ac.uk

The Role of Clinical Pathways in Reducing the Economic Burden of Stroke

Douglas J. Lanska

Tomah Veterans Affairs Medical Center, Great Lakes VA Health Care System, Tomah, Wisconsin, USA, and Department of Neurology, University of Wisconsin, Madison, Wisconsin, USA

The search for management and oversight strategies to optimise the use of healthcare resources has been driven by rapidly escalating healthcare costs, intense competitive pressures and a growing suspicion that a large proportion of the healthcare provided is either inappropriate or inefficient. In particular, the recognition of large geographical differences in resource use within the US has raised difficult questions about whether these differences reflect unnecessary costs in high-use areas, less than optimal care in low-use areas or some combination of the two.[1] With regard to stroke, for example, there are large geographical differences in the duration of hospital stay in the US, with average durations of stay in the northeast of up to 6 days longer than in other areas of the country.[2] While the duration of hospital stay for stroke has been declining since the 1960s, the absolute differentials in duration of stay between geographical regions have remained relatively constant over the past 30 years.[2]

Because of intense pressures to reduce healthcare costs, many organisations have sought management strategies to reduce resource use while maintaining the quality of care. In most cases, this has involved an increased scrutiny of hospital admissions as well as increased scrutiny of expensive technologies and treatments (e.g. utilisation review and quality assurance programmes), combined with standardisation and optimisation of the process of medical care (e.g. practice parameters, clinical pathways, continuous quality improvement and case management).

1. Clinical Pathways

Clinical pathways are one common management strategy for both improving healthcare efficiency and decreasing costs, while also maintaining, or ideally improving, quality of care. Clinical pathways are condition-specific multidisciplinary patient care management plans, which generally specify discipline-specific responsibilities, specific interventions and a specific sequence or timing of services intended to achieve specified patient care goals with optimal efficiency. Among other things, clinical pathways may incorporate standard admission orders, documentation requirements, and transfer and discharge criteria. Regardless of the exact pathway components, 'variances' – i.e. deviations from the pathway that might alter the anticipated discharge date, expected costs or expected outcomes – are routinely monitored so that system inefficiencies can be identified and corrected.

Although relatively few clinical pathways for stroke have been described in the medical literature,[3-9] and although the reported benefits have been mixed, more and more hospitals are adopting clinical pathways as a management strategy for patients with stroke. Indeed, in a recent survey, 14 of 187 (7%) hospitals that responded were currently using or were developing stroke clinical pathways.[10] Further application of this technology to stroke can be expected, in part because of support from healthcare leaders and national medical groups.[11] Indeed, some of the participants at a recent National Symposium on Rapid Identification and Treatment of Acute Stroke concluded that all hospitals treating patients with acute stroke should develop a stroke plan that incorporates available evidence-based practice guidelines into institution-specific algorithms and clinical pathways.[11] In particular, emergency departments were encouraged to have specialised protocols or clinical pathways in place to ensure provision of recombinant tissue plasminogen activator (rTPA) or other critically time-dependent agents to eligible patients within a narrow therapeutic time window.[11]

Some stroke clinical pathways focus on acute care for stroke,[4,6-9] while others deal with inpatient rehabilitation.[3,5] Descriptions of the pathways are at best sketchy in most of the published reports, although more detailed supplementary materials are available in some cases.[3,6] Components of most acute stroke pathways include the following:

- standard admission orders
- early evaluation of dysphagia (usually on day 1 or 2)
- early involvement of allied health personnel (including physical therapists, occupational therapists, speech-language therapists and social workers – all usually on day 2)
- early involvement of physiatrists, if indicated
- early discharge planning (usually by day 3 or 4).

1.2 Differentiation from Critical Pathways

Clinical pathways are not identical to 'critical pathways,' although the terms are often inappropriately considered to be synonyms. Critical-path analysis (CPA), the critical-path method (CPM) and the programme-evaluation and review technique (PERT) are all terms for sophisticated analytical tools developed in the 1950s and 1960s to plan and manage both industrial production processes and complicated research and development projects.[12] The PERT technique, for example, was first developed in the late 1950s by the US Naval Special Projects Office and applied to the development of the Polaris nuclear submarine.[13]

All of these so-called 'project network techniques' involve the diagrammatic representation of the individual steps in a complex task or project. The diagram takes the form of a specialised flow chart or 'network flow diagram,' which pictorially illustrates the sequential and interrelated activities and events in the project.[12-14] Events are specific points in the progress of a project, and activities are the procedures that must be performed to progress from event to event.[12,13]

Once a complete network flow diagram is constructed, the time required to complete each activity is estimated. Activity times are derived or estimated from historical data in somewhat different ways for different project network techniques: for example, CPM uses the average activity time as an estimate, while PERT uses a variety of estimates from worst case to best case to derive an 'expected' activity time. In any case, it is important to note that these times are not just the times required for the direct labour involved in the activities, but rather represent the entire time to schedule and complete the activities or achieve the desired outcomes.

The 'critical path' through a network is the particular sequence of activities which determines the total time for the task, i.e. the pathway from the starting point to the ending point that takes (or is expected to take) the longest amount of time. If the overall time for completion of a complex activity is to be shortened, some portion of the critical path will need to be changed. The benefit of project network techniques is precisely that they allow the identification of the critical activities so that these particular activities may be carefully scrutinised and, if necessary, altered to shorten the total project time. Of course, in reducing the times of the initial critical activities, new critical pathways may be created which must then be similarly scrutinised until the entire process is optimised. Reductions in the critical path can be obtained by:

- eliminating redundant or unnecessary activities
- shortening specific activity times (e.g. by changing procedures, decreasing waiting times, etc.)
- overlapping certain activities
- increasing the resources employed (e.g. by transferring resources from noncritical to critical activities).

Unfortunately, the formal project network techniques used in industry have not yet been applied in clinical medicine to change the processes of care,[14] although they have been used in the design and control of a complex medical research project.[13] Nevertheless, project network techniques hold great promise for improving the processes of medical care, particularly in terms of optimising the efficiency of inpatient hospital stays for common conditions such as stroke. The process of constructing a network flow diagram by itself could enhance understanding of the relationships between various activities and events in the care process. Moreover, the process of estimating activity times and determining the critical path will appropriately focus attention on the sequence of rate-limiting activities in the care process and allow targeted efforts to reduce the overall duration of hospital stay. An opportunity exists to apply this technology to acute care hospitalisations for stroke, and particularly to the emergency room evaluation and treatment of patients with acute ischaemic strokes of recent onset, so as to allow treatment of eligible patients with critically time-dependent therapies within a narrow therapeutic window.

2. Potential Benefits of Clinical Pathways

Even without the use of sophisticated project network techniques, clinical pathways have a number of potential benefits (see table I). Unfortunately, most of these anticipated benefits have yet to be documented in any trial of clinical pathways. Nevertheless, in published clinical pathways for acute stroke, the following benefits have been reported:

- reduced use of expensive diagnostic studies

Table I. Potential benefits of clinical pathways

Reduced variation in management practices
Identification of key clinical decision points
Increased collaboration and communication among caregivers
Elimination of system breakdowns
More specific and relevant chart documentation
Decreased use of expensive diagnostic tests
More appropriate use of treatment modalities
Fewer complications
Better control of liability risks
Reduced duration of hospital stay
Reduced patient charges
Better functional outcomes
Improved patient understanding and satisfaction with care
Greater frequency of return to independent living
Lower mortality

Table II. Reported benefits of clinical pathways for stroke

Reference (year)	Setting	Study design	Results								
			use of diagnostic studies	use of treatment modalities	incidence of complications	duration of stay	patient charges	functional status	patient satisfaction	nursing home placement	mortality
Romito[3] (1990)	Rehab	Uncontrolled	NA	NA	NA	ND	NA	NA	ND	NA	NA
Odderson & McKenna[4] (1993)	Acute	Historical controls	NA	NA	↓[a]	↓	↓	NA	NA	↔	↔
Falconer et al.[5] (1993)	Rehab	Randomised	NA	NA	NA	↔	↔	↔	↓	↔	↔
Bowen & Yaste[6] (1994)	Acute	Historical and concurrent controls	↑[b]	↑[c]	[d]	↓	↓	NA	NA	↔	↔
Duryee et al.[8] (1996)	Acute	Historical controls	↓[e]	NA	↔	↓	NA	NA	NA	NA	↓
Ramachandran et al.[9] (1996)	Acute	Historical controls	↓[f]	NA	ND	↓	ND	NA	NA	NA	↓

a Decreased urinary tract infections.
b Increased use of carotid ultrasound.
c Increased use of heparin prophylaxis for deep venous thrombosis.
d Complications were similar, including deep venous thrombosis, pneumonia, aspiration pneumonia and unspecified bacterial infections. Urinary tract infections were significantly decreased compared with only 1 control group.
e Decreased duplicate physical therapy evaluations.
f Decreased use of magnetic resonance imaging (MRI).
Acute = acute care hospital stay; **NA** = not assessed; **ND** = not adequately documented; **Rehab** = rehabilitation hospital stay; ↔ = no change; ↓ = decreased; ↑ = increased.

- fewer complications (particularly the frequency of urinary tract infections and aspiration pneumonia)
- reduced duration of hospital stay
- reduced patient charges
- lower mortality.

However, these reported benefits are not consistent across all studies (table II), and some of the outcomes are very highly correlated (e.g. duration of hospital stay and patient charges).

The most consistently reported benefit of stroke clinical pathways is a decrease in duration of hospital stay for acute stroke. Because clinical pathways focus on improving efficiency, this is not necessarily surprising. However, with the exception of the study by Bowen and Yaste,[6] which used both historical and concurrent controls, all of the studies documenting a decrease in the duration of stay were based on comparisons with historical controls.[4,8,9] Because the duration of hospital stay has been declining rather precipitously even without the implementation of clinical pathways,[2] it is not clear that the declines are necessarily attributable to the institution of clinical pathways.

Because duration of hospital stay and patient charges are generally highly correlated, it might be anticipated that patient charges are also generally lower with decreased duration of stay even when charges were not assessed or documented. Indeed, where decreased charges have been documented, it appears that a decrease in the duration of stay was a major contributor. However, in all of the available studies, charges were limited to acute care hospitalisation, so it is not clear whether some of the costs were merely shifted from inpatient to outpatient settings. Moreover, Pearson et al.[15] have argued that, 'Improvements [including decreases in duration of stay and patient charges] that some authors have attributed to critical pathways could have been achieved just as easily by simply instructing clinicians to manage patients within a specified target duration of stay'. Therefore, these reported benefits of clinical pathways should be considered tentative pending further studies.

To date, there is no clinical or scientific consensus on many aspects of stroke management. By themselves, clinical pathways will not fill the outstanding gaps in medical knowledge. However, by focusing attention on important aspects of care for which there is as yet no accepted best practice, clinical pathways may stimulate targeted studies, clinical consensus or evidence-based guidelines that can be incorporated into clinical algorithms.

3. Implementation Issues

Clinical pathways are clearly not a panacea: clinical pathways will most certainly not solve all issues and problems related to patient management. On the heels of considerable hype and fanfare, recognition of the difficulties associated with developing and implementing clinical pathways, and cognizance of the limitations of the final product, have often led to frustration and disillusionment. Indeed, as noted by Pearson et al.,[15] 'Hundreds of pathways created by flourishing programs fell quickly into disuse and even disregard, despite their early success . . .. Although the promise of reduced costs and improved quality is enticing, the gaps in our knowledge about critical pathways are extensive . . . . Therefore, like any new healthcare technology, pathway programs should be fully evaluated in order to understand the conditions under which that promise may be fulfilled . . .'.

In part, the high failure rate for clinical pathways is due to failures of planning and implementation. These facets have in fact been troubled by a large number of shortcomings, including the following: (i) lack of administrative and medical staff leadership; (ii) lack of multidisciplinary involvement; (iii) clinician resistance; (iv) failure to formulate and articulate quality and cost goals; (v) inadequate resources; (vi) unrealistic time frames; (vii) unnecessary added paperwork and documentation; (viii) burdensome variance reporting procedures; and (ix) a failure to cover the entire episode of care rather than just a hospital component.

In particular, adoption of clinical pathways by an institution does not ensure that these clinical pathways will be followed by clinicians. Common clinician concerns about clinical pathways – which must be overcome for successful implementation – are shown in table III. Changing physician behaviours is notoriously difficult, but behavioural change may be facilitated by education and appropriate feedback and by allowing physicians to participate in the development of clinical pathways and other change efforts. In some cases, administrative rules, financial incentives and even financial penalties may also be required.

Even with physician buy-in and co-operation, hospital efficiency may not be optimised until the pre- and post-hospitalisation aspects of care are optimised. For example, in a study by Goldman et al.,[16] delays while awaiting rehabilitation or other placement con-

Table III. Common clinician concerns about clinical pathways

Will erode physician autonomy
Are overly simplistic and rigid, giving a cookbook approach to medical care
Will restrict professional judgement
Variance data will be misused to judge competence/performance
Demonstrate no proven benefit for patient outcomes, and excessive emphasis on efficiency and costs may even potentially worsen health outcomes
Will increase malpractice risks
Will undermine teaching/research mission of hospitals

tributed the most unnecessary days of hospital care for patients with acute stroke (table IV). Such delays are generaly beyond the direct control of an institution that is endeavouring to implement a clinical pathway to optimise a hospital component of care. Creative solutions to overcome these obstacles may include the use of home healthcare and ambulatory rehabilitation services. However, reducing hospital costs by shifting these or greater costs to the outpatient setting does not produce true cost savings or other benefits, either for patients or the healthcare system.[15] Indeed, it is quite possible that true cost savings may only be achieved when the process of care is optimised across an integrated healthcare system.

Table IV. Reasons for unjustified hospital stay for 33 patients with acute stroke found by a consensus of neurologist reviewers to have more than 1 unnecessary day of hospitalisation

Type of delay	No. of cases (%)
Rehabilitation placement	15 (45)
Other placement	3 (9)
Testing	8 (24)
Consultation	5 (15)
Treatment	3 (9)
Other	5 (15)

4. Integration with Other Management Strategies

Clinical pathways by themselves will never be adequate to solve all of our healthcare financing or quality dilemmas, nor for that matter will any other available management strategy. Instead, optimal use of healthcare resources, control of escalating healthcare costs and improved quality of medical care will undoubtedly require a thoughtful combination of management strategies that integrates the best features of each into an overall coordinated programme.

For example, clinical pathway programmes are largely complementary to both utilisation review and case management programmes. Utilisation review programmes evaluate the appropriateness of hospitalisation and the use of expensive technologies.[17,18] In cases where utilisation is deemed inappropriate, such programmes act to restrict either utilisation itself or the reimbursement for such utilisation. These programmes thus meet different needs from those met by clinical pathways, which address 'the quality and efficiency of care *after* decisions have already been made to admit the patient or perform the procedure'.[15] Similarly, although both clinical pathway and case management programmes seek to improve system efficiency, critical pathways concentrate on high-volume conditions with high costs in which care is generally patternable, whereas case management focuses on low-volume conditions with high costs in which care is complex and not patternable.

Clinical pathways have also been integrated with and used to support quality assurance programmes. Quality assurance programmes evaluate the quality of care provided, generally by reviewing selected patient records. A subset of records may be chosen at random for review, or records may be selected on the basis of outcomes associated with a higher frequency of quality problems (e.g. drug toxicity, surgical complications, death, etc.). In cases where care is deemed by the review to be substandard, the programmes act to censure the responsible parties. While not an ideal approach for improving the quality of care, quality assurance programmes are needed to identify egregious deviations from quality medical care: as noted by Berwick,[19] 'Politically, at least, it is absolutely necessary for regulators to continue to ferret out the truly avaricious and the dangerously incompetent.'

Because variances from clinical pathways are routinely monitored to identify system inefficiencies, they are readily available and may also be scrutinised for quality problems. However, because physicians often perceive quality assurance programmes as adversarial, punitive, arbitrary and burdensome,[20] the use of variance data for quality assurance purposes may be counterproductive in terms of eliciting physician trust and cooperation (see section 3).

Clinical pathways have also occasionally been integrated with continuous quality improvement programmes, as for example in refinement of protocols for reduction of delays between emergency department admission and treatment of acute stroke,[21] but this is an area that warrants much greater emphasis. In contrast to quality assurance programmes, continuous quality improvement programmes attempt to shift the process of care for all providers and not just the outliers.

If carefully designed and implemented, and if properly viewed as a hypothesis of the best management strategy to be continuously evaluated and modified when necessary, clinical pathways can be an exemplar of the continuous quality improvement process. However, as noted by Marder,[22] 'If pathways simply catalog current standard orders without considering the sequencing of those orders, the only accomplishment might well be no more than the standardisation of inefficiencies . . . . If pathways are viewed as unmodifiable on a case-by-case basis and nurses or other case managers are placed in the position of gatekeepers, the pathways will contribute only conflict and tension . . . . If pathways focus narrowly on isolated tasks and are viewed as finished products rather than as opportunities for continuous improvement, then today's pathway based on current practices and standards will become tomorrow's outdated cookbook recipe . . .' Clinical pathways should be re-evaluated and modified when medical knowledge advances, when new practice parameters are developed,[17,18] when local conditions change or when improved clinical pathways are identified at other organisations.

5. Conclusion

Clinical pathways are a potentially beneficial, but largely untested, management strategy for both improving healthcare efficiency and decreasing costs while also maintaining or improving quality of care. Effective implementation of clinical pathways requires the following: (i) strong administrative and medical staff leadership; (ii) active participation of all clinical disciplines involved in the care of patients on the pathway; (iii) provision of regular feedback to clinicians on quality and cost goals, compliance, variances and outcomes; (iv) sufficient resources (including people, time and money); (v) improved documentation including simple and efficient charting and variance reporting procedures; (vi) incorporation of the entire episode of care into the pathway rather than just a hospital component; (vii) integration of the clinical pathway development and implementation process with ongoing quality and utilisation management programmes; and (viii) periodic evaluation and modification of the clinical pathway if necessary.

Although not yet truly implemented in clinical medicine, formal project network techniques, such as CPA and the programme evaluation and review technique, hold great promise for improving the processes of medical care, particularly in terms of optimising the efficiency of inpatient hospital stays for common conditions such as stroke.

References

1. Epstein AM. The outcomes movement: will it get us where we want to go? N Engl J Med 1990; 323: 266-70
2. Lanska DJ. Length of stay for patients admitted with stroke in the United States: Professional Activity Study, 1963-1991. J Neurol Sci 1994; 127: 214-20
3. Romito D. A critical path for CVA patients. Rehabil Nurs 1990; 15: 153-6
4. Odderson IR, McKenna BS. A model for management of patients with stroke during the acute phase: outcome and economic implications. Stroke 1993; 24: 1823-7
5. Falconer JA, Roth EJ, Sutin JA, et al. The critical path method in stroke rehabilitation: lessons from an experiment in cost containment and outcome improvement. Qual Rev Bull 1993; 19: 8-16
6. Bowen J, Yaste C. Effect of a stroke protocol on hospital costs of stroke patients. Neurology 1994; 44: 1961-4
7. Hydo B. Designing an effective clinical pathway for stroke. Am J Nurs 1995; 95 (3): 44-50
8. Duryee R, Calanchini P, Miller R. The impact of a stroke clinical pathway: measuring effectiveness [abstract]. Neurology 1996; 46: A428
9. Ramachandran TS, Culebras A, Hainsworth D. Development and implementation of a clinical pathway for stroke in acute care [abstract]. Neurology 1996; 46: A319
10. Anderson Consulting. Clinical path survey: a study of clinical path trends in healthcare. Dallas (TX): Anderson Consulting, 1995
11. Setting new directions for stroke care: proceedings of National Symposium on Rapid Identification and Treatment of Acute Stroke. Bethesda (MD): National Institute of Neurological Disorders and Stroke, 1997
12. Lockyer K, Gordon J. Critical path analysis and other project network techniques. 5th ed. London: Pitman Publishing, 1991
13. Woolf CR, Cass W, McElroy J. The use of 'program evaluation and review technique' (PERT) in the design and control of a medical research project. Comput Biomed Res 1968; 2: 176-86
14. Luttman RJ, Laffel GL, Pearson SD. Using PERT/CPM to design and improve clinical processes. Qual Manage Health Care 1995; 3 (2): 1-13
15. Pearson SD, Goulart-Fisher D, Lee TH. Critical pathways as a strategy for improving care: problems and potential. Ann Intern Med 1995; 123: 941-8
16. Goldman RS, Hartz AJ, Lanska DJ, et al. Results of a computerized screening of stroke patients for unjustified hospital stay. Stroke 1996; 27: 639-44
17. Lanska DJ and the Task Force on Hospital Utilization for Stroke, American Academy of Neurology. Review criteria for hospital utilization for patients with cerebrovascular disease. Neurology 1994; 44: 1531-2
18. Lanska DJ. A public/private partnership in the quest for quality: development of cerebrovascular disease practice guidelines and review criteria. Am J Med Qual 1995; 10: 100-6
19. Berwick DM. Continuous improvement as an ideal in health care. N Engl J Med 1989; 320: 53-6
20. Lanska DJ. Medicare hospital utilization review for ischemic cerebrovascular disease. Neurology 1993; 43: 650-4
21. Tilley BC, Lyden PD, Brott TG, et al. Total quality improvement method for reduction of delays between emergency department admission and treatment of acute ischemic stroke. Arch Neurol 1997; 54: 1466-74
22. Marder RJ. The interface of clinical paths and continuous quality improvement. In: Spath PL, editor. Clinical paths: tools for outcomes management. Chicago (IL): American Hospital Publishing Inc., 1994: 57-78

Correspondence: Dr *Douglas J. Lanska*, Veterans Affairs Medical Center, 500 E. Veterans Street, Tomah, WI 54660, USA.

Thrombolysis, Stroke Units and Other Strategies for Reducing Acute Stroke Costs

Theodore H. Wein, *Susan L. Hickenbottom* and *Andrei V. Alexandrov*

Department of Neurology, University of Texas – Houston Medical School, Houston, Texas, USA

Stroke is the leading cause of long term disability in North America; there are an estimated 3 million stroke survivors in the US.[1] In 1992, the American Heart Association (AHA) estimated that there were 500 000 new cases of stroke annually in the US, and as the third leading cause of death after cancer and heart disease, stroke accounted for approximately 150 000 deaths per year.[1] Currently, stroke accounts for almost 1% of hospital admissions in the US, and approximately 140 000 individuals are transferred to nursing homes each year following non-fatal stroke. The total cost for stroke, consisting of both direct healthcare expenses and indirect personal financial loss, has been estimated at $US40.9 billion per year (1997 values).[1,2] The AHA recently reported that a stroke care expenditure of $US26.2 billion was the result of hospital care, professional care and medications while $US14.7 billion was accounted for by indirect costs such as lost labour (1997 values). In a prior study in 1994, it was estimated that the mean lifetime cost per person from ischaemic stroke was $US90 981. Indirect costs (rehabilitation, long term care, lost wages) have been estimated to account for 56 to 58% of total lifetime expenses.[3] More recent studies have reported direct healthcare expenditures of $US17 billion per year and estimated total stroke expenses at $US40 billion per year (1997 values)[3] with a mean lifetime cost per person of $US90 981 for ischaemic stroke (1994 values).[4,5] Indirect costs have been estimated to account for 56 to 58% of total lifetime expenses.[6,7]

After initial hospitalisation, rehabilitation and nursing homes account for the majority of stroke-related costs.[8] Acute care costs for first stroke account for 45% of total lifetime accrued stroke-related expenses in both the US and the Netherlands.[6,7] Jørgensen et al.[9] estimated that 93% of direct hospital costs for the treatment of stroke was accounted for by hospital overheads and nursing salaries. Smurawska et al.,[10] using a prevalence based study, established that nursing-related costs accounted for 42% of acute stroke care costs. Length of hospital stay (LOHS) is also a major determinant of total inpatient costs and accounts for 72 to 82% of the variation in inpatient costs.[11] Thus, along with reducing disability after stroke, cost-effective therapeutic interventions should:

- target and alter the LOHS
- increase the number of patients discharged to home
- decrease the number of individuals requiring inpatient or long term rehabilitation
- and diminish the need for nursing home placement.

The use of recombinant tissue plasminogen activator (rt-PA) for the treatment of acute ischaemic stroke and the implementation of stroke units (SU) are 2 recent developments which are proving useful in reaching these goals. According to Furlan,[12] acute stroke plans are designed to reduce management delays, maximise the potential number of thrombolytic candidates, minimise the number of stroke-related complications and improve outcome and decrease the LOHS. Therefore, the cost of rt-PA therapy, its implementation and specialised stroke care costs are closely interrelated.

The purpose of this review is to discuss the data on: (i) the effectiveness of rt-PA therapy to reduce disability after stroke; (ii) projected cost savings with and implementation of rt-PA therapy; and (iii) advantages of specialised care delivery through stroke units and acute stroke plans. We review these topics because the success and cost effectiveness of rt-PA therapy delivery is only possible with rational resource utilisation and stroke expertise as well as implementation of clinical pathways and quality improvement.[12] The delivery of specialised multilevel stroke care from the emergency room to rehabilitation should help realise cost savings for all patients who have had a stroke, whether or not they receive rt-PA.

1. Thrombolysis for Acute Ischaemic Stroke

1.1 Effectiveness of Thrombolytic Therapy

Several randomised, placebo-controlled trials have evaluated intravenous thrombolysis with streptokinase and rt-PA for acute ischaemic stroke (table I). A favourable outcome was observed in only 1 trial; in this trial, rt-pA 0.9 mg/kg was administered.[18] Outcomes were unfavourable in the trials of streptokinase because of high rates of intracerebral haemorrhage (ICH) and mortality (19 to 43%). A prior trial of rt-PA at a higher dose of 1.1 mg/kg showed a 20% ICH rate but no significant difference in mortality.[8,13-18] Based on the results of the National Institute of Neurological Disorders and Stroke (NINDS) study (table I), the US FDA in June of 1996 approved the use of rt-PA in a dose of 0.9 mg/kg as the first, and so far only, therapy for acute ischaemic stroke in a select group of patients i.e. those who can be treated within 3 hours of symptom onset. Part I of the NINDS trial assessed outcomes at 24 hours in 291 patients, and Part II assessed outcomes at 3 months in 333 patients.

In Part I, no significant difference between patients treated with rt-PA versus placebo was found.[8] However, it did reveal a trend towards early improvement or return to normal function in 47% of thrombolytic-treated patients as compared with 39% of patients who received placebo at 24 hours. While this trend did not reach statistical significance, it is important to note that one of the investigators' prespecified end-points was defined as an improvement by 4 or more points on the National Institute of Health Stroke Scale (NIHSS). Review of the data reveals that the median NIHSS score in the rt-PA-treated group was 14 at baseline and 8 at 24 hours. In contrast, in the placebo group, the NIHSS score was 14 at baseline and 12 at 24 hours ($p < 0.02$). Thus, it is likely that a positive effect of rt-PA does exist at 24 hours.

Part II of the study used several outcome scales to assess independence and functionality at 3 months. An 11 to 13% absolute increase was found in the number of rt-PA-treated patients classified as having minimal or no disability as measured by the Barthel Index, modified Rankin Scale, NIHSS and Glasgow Outcome Scale as compared with placebo recipients. Thus, patients treated with rt-PA were at least 30% more likely to have minimal or no disability at 3 months. The outcomes included a symptomatic ICH rate of 6.4% in the thrombolytic group

Table I. Randomised placebo-controlled trials of intravenous thrombolysis for ischemic stroke

Study	Drug/dose	Treatment window (h)	BP parameters	Favourable outcome[a]	ICH[b] rate (%)	Death and comments
NINDS[18]	rt-PA 0.9 mg/kg	<3	SBP < 185mm Hg; DPB < 110mm Hg	Yes	6.4	Mortality: 17% (rt-PA) *vs* 21% (placebo)
ECASS[13,14]	rt-PA 1.1 mg/kg	<6	No	No, see comments	19.0	Mortality: 19.4% (rt-PA) *vs* 14.8% (placebo). Significant secondary end-points[c]
ECASS II[19]	rt-PA 0.9 mg/kg	<6	SBP < 185mm Hg; DBP < 110 mm Hg	No	8.8	Mortality 10.5% (rt-PA) *vs* 10.7% (placebo)
MAST-I[15]	SK 5×10^6U + AS 300mg	<6	No	No	6.0	10-day mortality: 27% (SK + AS) *vs* 12% (placebo). Study stopped early secondary to high ICH and mortality
MAST-E[16]	SK 1.5×10^6U	<6	No	No	17.5	10-day mortality: 35% (SK) *vs* 18% (placebo). Study stopped early secondary to high ICH and mortality
ASK[17,18]	SK 1.5×10^6U	<4	No	No	13.0	90-day mortality 43% (SK) *vs* 22% (placebo). Study stopped early secondary to high ICH and mortality

a Asymptomatic or minimal disability.

b Symptomatic ICH or parenchymal haematoma. Different criteria were used in each study.

c At 90 days, 41% of the rt-PA group [the target population (i.e. not intention-to-treat) rt-PA group] had asymptomatic or minimal disability (modified Rankin 0 or 1) *vs* 29% of placebo recipients.

AS = aspirin [acetylsalicylic acid]; **ASK** = Australian Streptokinase Trial; **BP** = blood pressure; **DBP** = diastolic blood pressure; **ECASS** = European Cooperative Acute Stroke Study; **ECASS II** = Second European-Australasian Acute Stroke Study; **ICH** = intracerebral haemorrhage; **MAST-E** = Multicentre Acute Stroke Trial – Europe; **MAST-I** = Multicentre Acute Stroke Trial – Italy; **NINDS** = National Institute of Neurological Disorders and Stroke; **rt-PA** = recombinant tissue plasminogen activator; **SBP** = systolic blood pressure; **SK** = streptokinase; **U** = units.

and 0.6% in the placebo group ($p < 0.001$). Despite the higher ICH rate with thrombolytic therapy, no difference in mortality was found between the 2 groups (17% rt-PA *vs* 21% placebo; not significant) at 3 months.[8,20]

The Second European-Australasian Acute Stroke Study (ECASS II) evaluated rt-PA in a dose of 0.9 mg/kg administered up to 6 hours from onset of symptoms.[19] In this study, the results did not demonstrate a statistical benefit for rt-PA although there was a trend towards efficacy particularly in patients who were treated early (< 3 hours). The ECASS trialists concluded that despite the increased risk of ICH (8.8 *vs* 3.4%), rt-PA in a dose of 0.9 mg/kg in selected patients (< 3 hours) may lead to a clinically relevant improvement in outcome. There was no difference in mortality (10.5 *vs* 10.7%)

With regard to intra-arterial thrombolysis, preliminary data from the Prolyse in Acute Cerebral Thromboembolism Trial (PROACT) trial of pro-urokinase in patients with acute ischaemic stroke showed favourable angiographic recanalisation rates. However, no data are yet available regarding patient outcomes.[21] A pilot study by Lanzieri et al.[22] showed that urgent intra-arterial thrombolysis with urokinase would result in a direct medical/treatment cost increase of $US1724 per patient (1995 values) treated. This increase was not significant when compared with patients who received standard stroke care [$US15 202 (group treated with thrombolysis) vs $US13 478 (standard care/no thrombolysis)]. The authors found a 5.12 point improvement of the NIHSS in patients treated with intra-arterial urokinase (n = 8) versus standard stroke therapy (n = 25, p = 0.0088). Intra-arterial thrombolysis reduced the number of completed stroke by 33% and fewer patients required admission to a nursing care facility. This resulted in a cost reduction of $US3435 from extended care institutions.

So far, no stroke thrombolysis regimen has met all 5 justification criteria for a new therapy as defined by Furlan and Kanoti.[23] These criteria include: 'safety', 'efficacy', 'effectiveness', 'efficiency' and 'outcome'. In section 1.2, we examine the data on the efficiency (or net benefit *vs* net cost) of intravenous rt-PA therapy based on the results of the NINDS study.

1.2 Projected Cost Savings with rt-PA Therapy

Fagan et al.[24] have recently conducted a cost benefit analysis of thrombolytic therapy with rt-PA by using a Markov model that estimated costs per 1000 patients eligible for thrombolytic treatment. This model explored the interaction between disability and dependency scores and the cost of drug therapy, prolonged intensive care monitoring and the risk of ICH. Primary health outcome was measured by the number of quality-adjusted life-years (QALYs) saved. This model assumed an average patient age of 67 years and estimated the cost of rt-PA as ranging from $US2100 to $US2400 per patient (1996 values). Drug monitoring costs were estimated at $US775 and complications with ICH were estimated to add an additional $US4500. The model also assumed that disability rates prior to the trial were similar in both placebo and rt-PA groups but did not take into account indirect costs such as loss of wages or work days lost. The investigators designed their model based on assumptions regarding stroke epidemiology, recovery, LOHS and costs (direct and indirect healthcare costs). These assumptions were drawn from the NINDS study and from literature review and are reproduced in table II.

A 1.5-day difference in LOHS was found in favour of the rt-PA-treated group with the average LOHS being 10.9 days in the thrombolytic group and 12.4 days in the placebo group (p = 0.02). In the treatment group, 48% of patients were discharged directly to home compared with 36% in the placebo cohort, and 14% fewer required inpatient rehabilitation or nursing home care (p = 0.002). In addition, this model predicted that in spite of an estimated 55 ICHs per 1000 patients treated, 116 more patients would have minimal or no disability and would subsequently be discharged directly to home if treated with rt-PA than with placebo (i.e. 316 *vs* 200 patients as projected if the NINDS data is applied to 1000 patients). Estimated additional costs for increased monitoring and management of ICH and other related complications were calculated at $US1700 per patient for patients treated with rt-PA. Given that 8.8 patients needed to be treated to discharge an additional patient home, an additional cost of $US15 000 would accrue in order for an additional patient to be discharged home instead of requiring nursing home placement or inpatient rehabilitation. This translates to a projected acute care and rehabilitation saving of $US600 000 per year per 1000 patients treated. While thrombolytic therapy would increase direct hospital costs of $US1.7 million per 1000 patients, reductions in costs of $US4.8 million for nursing homes and by $US1.3 million for rehabilitation would result one year following treatment.

Overall, this model predicts with a certainty of greater than 90% that a net savings will occur with rt-PA therapy. Finally, over a 30-year period, the Markov model predicts that 564 QALYs would be saved per 1000 patients. QALYs ranged from 765 to 335 when ICH rates were varied from 6 to 20%, and when the mortality factor was varied from 1.25 to 4, QALYs ranged from 1129 to 575.

Table II. Assumptions by NINDS investigators[24]

Patient care costs (ascending order) and LOHS	Low	Best	High
Nursing home cost per year ($US)	20 000	39 996	50 000
Inpatient rehabilitation cost ($US)	10 000	21 233	40 000
ICH additional cost ($US)	3 000	4 500	6 000
Outpatient rehabilitation cost ($US)	1 200	2 236	2 500
Average rt-PA acquisition cost ($US)	2 100	2 230	2 400
Cost per day of hospitalisation ($US)	1 000	1 200	1 400
ICU additional cost for patients treated with rt-PA ($US)	600	775	1 000
Physician cost for administration of rt-PA ($US)	200	300	400
Cost of preparation and administration of rt-PA ($US)	10	20	30
Average LOHS for patients treated with rt-PA (days)	9.7	10.88	12.0
Average LOHS for patients treated with placebo (days)	11.2	12.41	13.7

ICH = intracerebral haemorrhage; **ICU** = intensive care unit; **LOHS** = length of hospital stay; **NINDS** = National Institute of Neurological Disorders and Stroke; **rt-PA** = recombinant tissue plasminogen activator.

1.3 Implementation of rt-PA Therapy

Implementing rt-PA therapy within a 3-hour window from onset of symptoms poses a formidable challenge that can be, and has been, overcome. Rapid assessment of patients with potential stroke may be achieved by instituting a hyperacute stroke response team. Immediate notification about patients with a potential stroke by direct interaction and coordination with ambulance services and emergency department staff can alert stroke team members to potential thrombolytic candidates even prior to their arrival. By maximising available resources and preassigning and prioritising responsibilities of healthcare staff, clinical, laboratory and radiographic evaluations can be performed in an efficient manner to minimise the 'door-to-drug' time. The placement of rt-PA in the emergency department pharmacy or in a locked cabinet in the emergency room are additional time saving measures that may be easily implemented. A systematic approach to delivering thrombolytic therapy within a 55-minute window has recently been published by the NINDS investigators.[25] These investigators claim that a hyperacute stroke response system can be implemented at a minimal cost offset by the long term cost savings of using rt-PA.[25]

At the University of Texas at Houston, we have implemented many of these methods at no additional cost to the hospital (personal communication, Dr J.C. Grotta, Professor of Neurology, University of Texas, Houston, January 1998). However, this may not be feasible for other institutions. Furthermore, unavailability of urgent access to neuroimaging and specialised stroke monitoring units would preclude certain institutions from implementing acute stroke care plans.[12]

The use of intravenous rt-PA has generated much controversy regarding its safety, feasibility and cost. Many have argued that results from a clinical trial setting, in which patients are carefully selected, are not generalisable to actual practice. A former NINDS site reported its centre's 1-year experience after publication of the NINDS trial. Outcomes and complication rates were nearly identical to the NINDS Study.[26] Similar observations have been reported from other centres, including community hospitals.[27,28]

Thrombolytic therapy offers the possibility of reducing the severity of stroke, decreasing LOHS and theoretically diminishing the intensity of nursing care a patient requires, thus leading to cost savings. However, administration of rt-PA therapy as well as the overall diagnosis and management of stroke requires special training and a systematic approach. Therefore, the next question that needs to be addressed is whether implementation of specialised stroke care may also be beneficial in reducing LOHS and stroke-related costs; this is addressed in section 2.

2. Stroke Units

There is mounting evidence that treating all patients who have had a stroke in specialised SUs is beneficial in decreasing patient mortality, LOHS, and rehabilitation- and stroke-related costs. However, when reviewing the literature, one must pay careful attention to the nosology of the term, 'stroke unit,' because it may refer to: (i) a multidisciplinary team that follows patients on different floors of a hospital; (ii) a stroke team assigned to a dedicated stroke ward working exclusively with patients who have had an acute and/or subacute stroke with the goal of discharging patients within 7 to 10 days; (iii) an acute/subacute stroke care unit combined with rehabilitation facilities; and (iv) a dedicated stroke rehabilitation unit.

In a randomised controlled trial,[29] 130 patients with stroke who required hospital admission were stratified to receive either conventional stroke care or care by a multidisciplinary stroke team that followed stroke patients in different areas of the hospital. No significant benefit was found when patients were cared for by a mobile stroke team. Rønning and Guldvog[30] randomised patients with an acute stroke (symptoms present for <24 hours) to receive either standard care on a general medical ward (GMW) [n = 438] or to be assigned to a 10-bed SU (n = 364) managed by a multidisciplinary stroke team consisting of a neurologist, nurses trained in stroke-related issues, physiotherapists, a speech therapist and occupational therapists, all of whom met weekly to discuss patient treatment and care.[30] All patients treated in the SU followed a critical pathway regarding diagnostic evaluation and standard orders for rehabilitation therapy. Hyperglycaemia was aggressively treated if serum glucose levels exceeded 12 mmol/L, and body temperature greater than 38°C was treated with antipyretic agents. At 10 days, case mortality rates were significantly higher in patients treated in the GMW (15.1%) than in individuals treated in the SU (8.2%, p = 0.0019). Survival at 12 months was 70.6% in the SU group and 64.6% (p = 0.026) in individuals treated in a GMW. This benefit was also seen at 18 months with survival rates of 65.1% in patients treated in the SU and 58.0% (p = 0.026) in patients treated in the GMW. The greatest benefit was seen in patients admitted with a diagnosis of ICH. At 10 days, this group had a mortality rate of 24.5% in patients treated in the SU versus 51.6% in patients treated in the GMW (p = 0.004).[30]

Jørgensen et al.[31] compared a SU (n = 936) with both a general neurological ward (GNW) and a GMW (total n= 305) to which patients with a stroke were admitted within 2 weeks from the onset of their symptoms.[31] Outcomes were mortality rates, LOHS and number of individuals discharged to a nursing home. Although the study was not randomised (a selection bias may have occurred), the SU proved superior to both the GMW and the GNW on all outcomes measured. In comparison with both general wards, mortality rates were 21% lower in patients treated in the SU [odds ratio (OR): 0.5; 95% confidence interval (CI): 0.34 to 0.74; p < 0.01] and LOHS was reduced by 30% (p < 0.001). Discharge rates to home were significantly higher for patients treated in the SU (16%; OR: 1.9; 95% CI: 1.3 to 2.7; p < 0.001) than for those in the general wards whereas discharge rates to nursing homes were 20% lower (OR: 0.61; 95% CI: 0.38 to 0.98; p = 0.04). Patients treated in the SU had relative risk reductions of 50% for death and 40% for nursing home placement and almost double the relative chance of being discharged home. Hence, the SU saved lives, reduced LOHS, reduced the frequency of patients being discharged to nursing homes and reduced costs by 1313 bed days per 100 patients. The results of this nonrandomised study are concordant with other randomised SU trials.[32-37]

The development of a specialised stroke rehabilitation unit has also been shown to be beneficial. In a prospective randomised trial of 71 patients with severe stroke and poor prognosis, Kalra and Eade[36] found that individuals treated in an inpatient stroke rehabilitation unit had a greater chance of being discharged home (47 *vs* 19%; $p < 0.01$) as well as a decreased LOHS (43 *vs* 59 days; $p < 0.02$) when compared with patients treated in a GMW. Although inpatient rehabilitation may improve outcome, it comes at the expense of increased LOHS. Since many hospitals in Europe and Canada include inpatient rehabilitation in stroke patient care, they usually report longer LOHS when compared with US hospitals which facilitate early discharge of these patients.[10,36] Functional outcome as measured by the Barthel Index revealed a trend towards higher scores in the SU group; however, this difference did not reach statistical significance.

A detailed report of stroke unit methodologies was published recently, in which the Stroke Unit Trialist Collaboration reported the results of a meta-analysis of 19 SU trials which included 3249 patients.[37] The analysts recontacted authors to provide some homogeneity to the data in order to account for the differences in SU definition, outcome measures and time of admission from the onset of symptoms. Median 1-year follow-up revealed death rates of 20.9% in patients treated in SUs and 25.4% in patients treated in GMWs (OR: 0.83; 95% CI: 0.69 to 0.98; $p < 0.05$). In other words, 22 patients need to be treated in a SU in order to prevent 1 death. A reduction in LOHS of 8% (95% CI: 3 to 13%) was documented for patients treated in SUs; however, there was marked heterogeneity in these results. The percentage of individuals unable to live at home was 40.1% in the SU group and 47.2% in the GMW group; therefore, 14 patients (range: 8 to 30) need to be treated in a SU for one to be able to live at home. 40% of patients treated in SUs were independent (able to live at home) at discharge compared with 33.6% of patients treated in GMWs, implying that 16 patients (range: 10 to 25) need to be treated in a SU in order for one to be independent.

Despite variations in methodologies, SU trials have shown consistent trends towards or significant reductions in mortality and LOHS and improvements in outcomes compared with the current standard of care (standard stroke treatemnt on a GMW). The reason why SUs are effective as yet remains unclear. SUs may result in improved patient outcome by promoting rapid and efficient institution of intensive therapy (prevention of secondary stroke and early systemic complications of stroke, and early enrolment in occupational therapy, physical therapy, speech therapy and rehabilitation). SUs also provide consistency in stroke care by utilising critical pathways and a coordinated multidisciplinary approach to continuous education and training.

The ability to apply results from clinical trials to a community practice is of vital importance. Wentworth and Atkinson[38] implemented an acute response stroke team and SU in a 250-bed community hospital. By establishing a stroke team and a SU, they were able to decrease the LOHS from 7.0 to 4.6 days and decrease hospital expenditure from $US14 076 to $US10 740, a reduction that translated into total savings of $US453 000 per year (1990 to 1994 values). This was compared with their expenditure prior to implementing a stroke team and a stroke unit.

3. Conclusion

The cost of stroke is largely determined by the LOHS and patient disposition, particularly the need for long term care. Intravenous rt-PA is the first therapy to effectively improve outcomes in patients with acute stroke presenting within 3 hours from the onset of symptoms. Intravenous rt-PA, as well as any other interventions for stroke, needs to be delivered as early as possible.

The benefits of rt-PA therapy are 2-fold. Firstly, rt-PA improves stroke outcome,[8] shortens LOHS and reduces nursing home costs which result in approximately $US4 to $US5 million saved per 1000 patients treated (1996 values).[24] Secondly, the routine use of rt-PA therapy will result in the implementation of the NINDS rt-PA treatment protocol, as well as a stroke response team and eventually SUs that will provide careful and consistent patient evaluation, treatment and rehabilitation. Currently, 8 to 9 patients need to be screened so that 1 can be treated with intravenous rt-PA.[26] All patients who have a stroke, whether or not they are eligible for rt-PA therapy, may benefit from having access to other treatment options to prevent further brain damage and subsequent strokes by being assessed and managed by a multidisciplinary team of specialists in stroke.[39]

Acknowledgements

We wish to thank Dr James Grotta for a thorough peer review and useful suggestions in preparation of this manuscript.

References

1. American Heart Association (AHA). 1992 heart and stroke facts. Dallas (TX): AHA, 1992
2. Lanska D, Kryscio R. Geographic distribution of hospitalization rates, case fatality and mortality from stroke in the United States. Neurology 1995; 45: 634-40
3. American Heart Association. Heart and stroke facts statistics: 1997 statistical supplement. Dallas (TX): American Heart Association, 1997
4. Matchar D, Duncan P. Cost of stroke. Stroke Clin Updates 1994; 5: 9-12
5. Dobkin B. The economic impact of stroke. Neurology 1995; 45 Suppl. 1: S6-9
6. Taylor TN, Davis PH, Torner JC, et al. Lifetime cost of stroke in the United States. Stroke 1996; 27: 1459-66
7. Bergman L, van der Meulen JHP, Limburg M, et al. Costs of medical care after first ever stroke in the Netherlands. Stroke 1995; 26: 1830-6
8. The National Institute of Neurological Disorders and Stroke rt-PA Stroke Study Group: tissue plasminogen activator for acute ischemic stroke. N Engl J Med 1995; 333: 1581-7
9. Jørgensen HS, Hirofumi N, Raaschou H, et al. Acute stroke care and rehabilitation: an analysis of the direct cost and its clinical and social determinants. Stroke 1997; 28: 1138-41
10. Smurawska LT, Alexandrov AV, Bladin CF, et al. Cost of acute stroke care in Toronto, Canada. Stroke 1994; 25: 1628-31
11. Holloway RG, Witter DM, Lawton KB, et al. Inpatient costs of specific cerebrovascular events at five academic medical centers. Neurology 1996; 46: 854-60
12. Furlan A. Rapid identification and treatment of acute stroke, a national symposium. Bethesda (MD): National Institutes of Health (NIH), 1997. NIH publication no.: 97-4239
13. Hacke W, Kaste M, Fieschi C, et al. Intravenous thrombolysis with recombinant tissue plasminogen activator for acute hemispheric stroke. JAMA 1995; 275: 1017-25
14. Hacke W, Toni D, Steiner T, et al. rt-PA in acute ischemic stroke: results from the ECASS three hour cohort [abstract]. Stroke 1997; 28: 272
15. Multicentre Acute Stroke Trial – Italy (MAST-I) Group. Randomised controlled trial of streptokinase, aspirin and combination of both in treatment of acute ischaemic stroke. Lancet 1995; 346: 1509-14
16. Multicenter Acute Stroke Trial – Europe (MAST-E) Study Group. Thrombolytic therapy with streptokinase in acute ischemic stroke. N Engl J Med 1996; 335: 145-50
17. Donnan G, Davis S, Chambers B, et al. Streptokinase for acute ischemic stroke with relationship to time of administration. JAMA 1996; 276: 961-6
18. Donnan G, Davis S, Chambers B, et al. Trials of streptokinase in severe acute ischaemic stroke. Lancet 1995; 345: 578-9
19. Hacke W, Kaste M, Fieschi C, et al. Randomized double blind placebo controlled trial of thrombolytic therapy with intravenous alteplase in acute ischaemic stroke (ECASS II). Lancet 1998; 352: 1245-51

20. Haley EC, Lewandowski C, Tilley BC, for the NINDS Stroke Study Group. Myths regarding the NINDS rt-PA stroke trial: setting the record straight. Ann Emerg Med 1997; 30: 676-82
21. Del Zoppo G, Higashida R, Furlan A, et al. PROACT: a phase II randomized trial of recombinant pro-urokinase by direct arterial delivery in acute middle cerebral artery stroke. Stroke 1998; 29: 4-11
22. Lanzieri C, Tarr R, Landis D, et al. Cost-effectiveness of emergency intraarterial intracerebral thrombolysis: a pilot study. Am J Neuroradiol 1995; 16: 1987-93
23. Furlan A, Kanoti G. When is thrombolysis justified in patients with acute ischemic stroke? A bioethical perspective. Stroke 1997; 28: 214-8
24. Fagan S, Morgenstern L, Petitta A, et al. Cost-effectiveness of tissue plasminogen activator for acute ischemic stroke. Neurology 1998; 50 (4): 883-9
25. The National Institute of Neurological Disorders and Stroke (NINDS) rt-PA Stroke Study Group. A systems approach to immediate evaluation and management of hyperacute stroke: experience at eight centers and implications for community practice and patient care. Stroke 1997; 28: 1530-40
26. Chiu D, Krieger D, Villar-Cordova C, et al. Intravenous tissue plasminogen activator for acute ischemic stroke: feasibility, safety and efficacy in the first year of clinical practice. Stroke 1998; 29: 18-22
27. Tanne D, Mansbach H, Verro P, et al. Intravenous rt-PA for stroke in clinical practice: a multicenter evaluation of outcome [abstract]. Stroke 1998; 29 (1): 288
28. Grond M, Rudolf J, Schmulling S, et al. Can the NINDS results be transferred into daily routine [abstract]? Stroke 1998; 29 (1): 288
29. Dauphinee SW, Shapiro S, Bass E, et al. A randomized trial of team care following stroke. Stroke 1984; 15(5): 864-72
30. Rønning O, Guldvog B. Stroke units versus general medical wards, I: twelve and eighteen month survival. A randomized, controlled trial. Stroke 1998; 29: 58-62
31. Jørgensen H, Nakayama H, Raaschou H, et al. The effect of a stroke unit: reduction in mortality, discharge rate to nursing home, length of hospital stay and cost. A community based study. Stroke 1995; 26: 1178-82
32. Indredavik B, Bakke F, Slørdahl S, et al. Stroke unit treatment improves long-term quality of life: a randomized controlled trial. Stroke 1998; 29: 895-9
33. Indredavik B, Bakke F, Solberg R, et al. Benefit of a stroke unit: a randomized controlled trial. Stroke 1991; 22: 1026-31
34. Rønning OM, Guldvog B. Stroke unit versus general medical wards, II: neurological deficits and activities of daily living. A quasi-randomized controlled trial. Stroke 1998; 29: 586-90
35. Kaste M, Palomäki H, Sarna S. Where and how should elderly stroke patients be treated. Stroke 1998; 26: 249-53
36. Kalra L, Eade J. Role of stroke rehabilitation units in managing severe disability after stroke. Stroke 1995; 26: 2031-4
37. Stroke Unit Trialist Collaboration. Collaborative systematic review of the randomised trials of organised inpatient (stroke unit) care after stroke. BMJ 1997; 314: 1151-9
38. Wentworth D, Atkinson R. Implementation of an acute stroke program decreases hospitalization costs and length of stay. Stroke 1996; 27: 1040-3
39. Morgenstern L, Grotta J. Ischemic cerebrovascular disease. In: Rakel R, editor. Conn's current therapy. Philadelphia (PA): W.B. Saunders, 1997: 881-8

Correspondence: Dr *Theodore Wein*, Stroke Team, Department of Neurology, University of Texas – Houston Medical School, 6431 Fannin, MSB. 7.044, Houston, Texas 77030, USA.
E-mail: twein@neuro.med.uth.tmc.edu

The Burden of Stroke and its Sequelae

Richard F. Gillum and *Jacqueline B. Wilson*

Centers for Disease Control and Prevention, Hyattsville, Maryland, USA

In 1993, the third leading cause of death in the US was cerebrovascular disease, following diseases of the heart and malignant neoplasms.[1] Stroke was also a leading cause of illness in the US, causing health expenditures in the thousands of millions of dollars.

This report examines the occurrence of stroke by age, sex, and race, and geographic area in the US population with special emphasis on persons 65 years of age and over. The utilisation of healthcare services for stroke, disability caused by stroke, and cost of illness attributable to direct costs and indirect costs are also considered.

Mortality data were derived from published and unpublished reports of the National Center for Health Statistics (NCHS).[2] Stroke was coded as the underlying cause of the deaths examined.[3] Population information was obtained for computation of death rates from published and unpublished data of the US Bureau of the Census for the US resident population. Data on characteristics of persons dying as a result of stroke were obtained from the National Mortality Follow-back Survey.[4]

It would be useful to obtain prevalence estimates from an examination survey in which medical history is corroborated by physical examination and medical records review. Unfortunately, the samples in the National Health Examination Survey and in the National Health and Nutrition Examination Surveys have been insufficient to provide reliable prevalence estimates. Therefore, the most valuable source of national prevalence data is the National Health Interview Survey (NHIS). Details of the survey methods have been published elsewhere.[5] In recent years, a one-sixth subsample of the NHIS sample responded to a check list of vascular diseases including the item 'Has anyone in the family ever had a stroke or a cerebrovascular accident?' To obtain more stable estimates, data for the 3 years 1990 to 1992 were combined.

Hospitalisation data were obtained from the National Hospital Discharge Survey,[6] a continuous survey since 1965. The data for the 1993 survey were obtained from the face sheets of a sample of inpatient medical records that were obtained from a national sample of short-stay general and specialty hospitals located in the US. Over 200 000 records from more than 400 hospitals were included. Numbers of discharges were examined with the principal (first-listed) diagnosis coded to stroke and its subcategories.[7] Hospital case fatality (the number of deaths divided by the number of total discharges multiplied by 100) was also examined. Further, the number of carotid endarterectomy (ICD9-CM 38.12) and carotid arteriography (ICD9-CM 88.41) procedures was enumerated. Population rates were computed using the US civilian population. Details of this survey have been published.[6]

Data on the utilisation of ambulatory care were obtained from the National Ambulatory

Medical Care Survey, a probability sample survey of office visits to nonfederally employed office-based physicians in 1994.[8] Data were obtained from patient encounter forms completed by participating physicians. Data on utilisation of nursing homes were obtained from the National Nursing Home Survey.[9,10] In these 2-stage probability samples, data on nursing home residents were obtained from interviews with nursing staff with access to the medical records. Data on 1995 personal healthcare expenditures were obtained from analyses of data from the Healthcare Financing Administration performed by Thomas A. Hodgson, PhD, the Chief Health Economist of the National Center for Health Statistics.

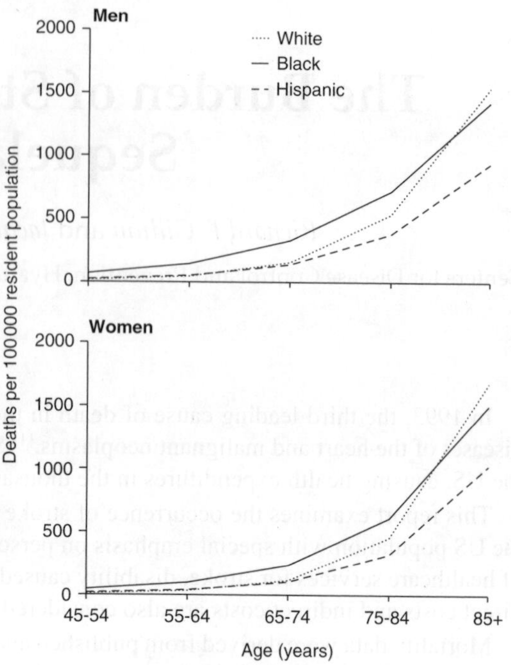

Fig. 1. Stroke death rates by race, Hispanic origin and age in men and women in 1989-91 (from Gillum,[12] with permission).

1. Mortality

1.1 Deaths

Of 2 268 553 deaths in 1993, 150 108 were attributed to stroke.[1] In 1992, cerebrovascular disease was the underlying cause of death in 143 769 cases but was mentioned on 255 418 death certificates.[11]

1.2 Age and Sex

Stroke mortality rates rose steeply with age in 1993 (fig. 1). Rates for the oldest age group must, however, be viewed with caution because of possible inaccuracies in reporting of age on death certificates relative to reporting age on census data. Age-adjusted stroke death rates per 100 000 were higher in men (29.0) than women (24.5) in 1993. Male to female ratios varied little with age in Whites (1.14 at ages 45 to 54 to 1.18 at age 75 to 84 years). In Blacks, the ratio declined from 1.40 at ages 45 to 54 to 1.21 at age 75 to 84 years.

1.3 Race

Stroke death rates were lower in Whites than Blacks in each age-sex group except for the 85+ group (fig. 1). The White-to-Black ratio increased with age in both sexes. However, these results for the oldest age group must be viewed with caution because of possible bias in age ascertainment.

1.4 Geographic Variation

An analysis was done of smoothed US stroke mortality rates per 100 000 by health service area. In White women aged 65 to 74 years in 1988 to 1992,[13,14] the highest rates were found in the East South Central Division followed closely by the southern South Atlantic, West South Central, and northern South Atlantic states. Surprisingly, rates were also high in the Pacific states. The lowest rates were found in the northern West North Central states and in New England. Patterns for age-adjusted rates were substantially similar. However, the pattern for ages 35 to 44 years revealed a more prominent cluster of relatively high rates west of the Mississippi River in the West South Central states. Rates were also high in the southern South Atlantic, Middle Atlantic and Pacific divisions.

In White men aged 65 to 74 years, the highest rates were found in the East South Central Division followed closely by the southern South Atlantic, West South Central and East North Central, northern South Atlantic states and Pacific states.[13,14] The lowest rates were found in the Mountain states. Patterns for age-adjusted rates were substantially similar. However, the pattern for ages 34 to 44 years revealed similar relatively high rates in the West South Central, southern South Atlantic, Middle Atlantic and Pacific divisions (map not shown). This pattern was similar to that in White women.

In an analysis of data from the National Center for Health Statistics from 1968 to 1985, the age-adjusted rate of death from stroke showed little effect of urbanisation in the Midwest and West.[14] However, in the Southeast and Northeast, death rates from stroke were higher in nonmetropolitan areas than in suburbs or central cities in both Whites and Blacks. Death rates were higher in the Southeast than in other regions for residents of small metropolitan and nonmetropolitan areas. A subsequent study of stroke incidence revealed higher incidence in the southeastern region of the US than in other regions.[15]

1.5 International Comparisons

Age-adjusted death rates for stroke in selected industrialised countries in 1990 reveal substantial variation.[16] Rates were high in Eastern Europe, intermediate in Western Europe and Japan, and lowest in North America. Variation in trends have also been reported with rapid declines in the English-speaking countries of North America and the Pacific and lesser declines or increases in Eastern Europe.[16]

1.6 Trends

For most of this century, death rates from stroke have declined in US Whites. Since 1960, the decline has been shared by all groups. With the rapid improvements in hypertension detection and control in the 1970s, the decline accelerated. Between 1979 and 1993, the long term decline in stroke mortality continued albeit at a slower rate than in the 1970s (table I).[16,17] Trends between 1979 and 1993 were downward in Whites and Blacks (table I). Black-to-White ratios increased slightly in men but showed no consistent change in women. Of considerable concern is the observation that death rates increased between 1992 and 1993, possibly heralding a pause in the long downward trend.

2. Morbidity

2.1 Prevalence

In the 1990 to 1992 National Health Interview Survey, it was estimated that 3.002 million persons in the civilian noninstitutionalised population had been diagnosed as having stroke

Table I. Age-adjusted death rates per 100 000 for cerebrovascular disease by sex and race: US 1950 to 1993 (from National Center for Health Statistics[2])

Year	White male	White female	Black male	Black female	Race ratio: male	Race ratio: female
1950	87.0	79.7	146.2	155.6	1.68	1.95
1960	80.3	68.7	141.2	139.5	1.76	2.03
1970	68.8	56.2	124.2	107.9	1.81	1.92
1980	41.9	35.2	77.5	61.7	1.85	1.75
1983	35.2	29.6	64.2	53.8	1.82	1.82
1984	33.9	28.9	62.8	51.8	1.85	1.79
1985	32.8	27.9	60.8	50.3	1.85	1.80
1986	31.1	27.1	58.9	47.6	1.89	1.76
1987	30.3	26.3	57.1	46.7	1.88	1.78
1988	30.0	25.5	57.8	46.6	1.93	1.83
1989	28.0	24.1	54.1	44.9	1.93	1.86
1990	27.7	23.8	56.1	42.7	2.03	1.79
1991	26.9	22.8	54.9	41.0	2.04	1.80
1992	26.3	22.5	52.0	39.9	1.98	1.77
1993	26.8	22.7	51.9	39.9	1.94	1.76

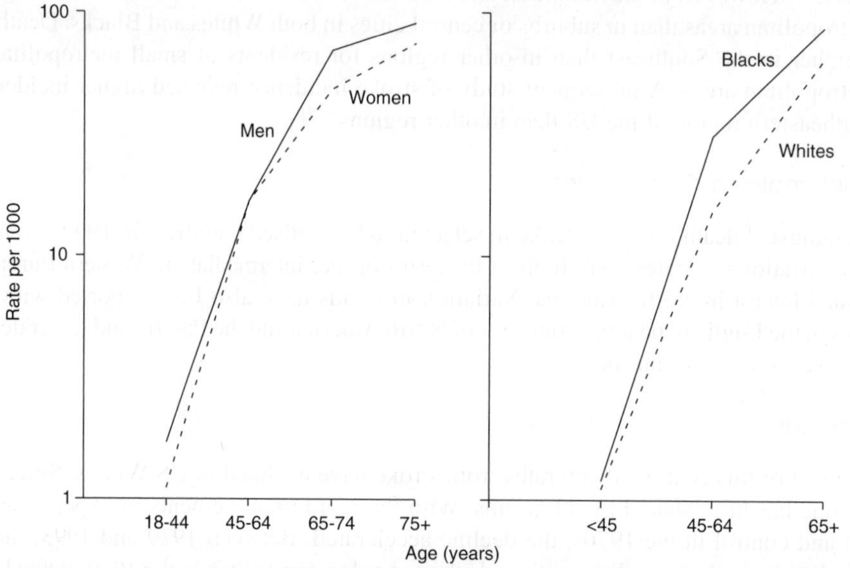

Fig. 2. Prevalence of self-reported stroke by sex (**left**) and race (**right**) in 1990 to 1992 (from National Health Interview Survey).

according to self-report.[18] The rate of stroke at age 65 to 74 years was 57.9 per 1000, rising to 80.8 at age 75 and over. The rate in elderly Whites aged 65 years and over (65.2 per 1000) was much lower than that in Blacks (87.8). Prevalence rates by age, sex and race in 1990 to 1992 are shown in figure 2. Rates were higher in Blacks than Whites at each age. An inverse relationship to income was apparent with higher rates for those with family income under $US10 000 compared with $US35 000 or more (table II). The self-reported prevalence rate at all ages was lowest in the Northeast region (9.3 per 1000) and highest in the South (14.5). The prevalence rate was higher in nonmetropolitan areas than in central cities or suburbs.

2.2 Hospitalisation

In 1993, 841 000 persons (629 000 aged 65 years of age and over) were discharged from short-stay nonfederal hospitals in the US with a first-listed diagnosis of stroke.[19,20] Of these, 274 000 had cerebral thrombosis or embolism (ICD9-CM 434) as the first-listed diagnosis (table III). The average length of stay was 8.4 days for all stroke patients. Over 2.65 million days of care were utilised by patients with first-listed diagnosis of cerebral thrombosis or embolism. Among persons 65 years and over, 1.365 million mentions of stroke occurred among the up to 7 diagnoses coded for each discharge. The rate of discharges with first-listed diagnosis of stroke was 1920 per 100 000 among persons 65 years and over in 1993. Among persons 65 and over, the hospital fatality rate was 7.8% for discharges with first-listed diagnosis of stroke (acute and chronic) compared with 5.4% for discharges under age 65.

Table II. Average annual number of self-reported stroke conditions, rate per 1000 persons by selected characteristics: US, 1990 to 1992 (from National Health Interview Survey)

Selected characteristic	Prevalence of conditions (thousands)	No. per 1000 persons
Total	**3002**[a]	**12.1**
Family income		
<$US10 000	601	24.8
$10 000 to 19 999	666	17.2
$20 000 to 34 999	558	10.6
≥$35 000	476	5.3
Region		
Northeast	466	9.3
Midwest	798	13.2
South	1225	14.5
West	513	9.5

a Includes unknown family income.

In view of the decline in stroke mortality in the elderly, an examination of trends in hospital discharge rate and hospital fatality rate is of interest. The hospital discharge rate for stoke in the elderly increased between 1980 and 1985 in both men and women but declined by 1988 with little further change (fig. 3).[21] Over the same period, the hospital fatality rate both in persons under 65 and 65 years and over decreased (fig. 4). A related phenomenon is the striking fluctuations in the rate of carotid endarterectomy procedures performed in persons 65 years and over between 1980 and 1992 (fig. 5).[21,22] These may relate to swings in opinion of physicians concerning the indications for the procedure.[22] Similarly the rate of inpatient carotid arteriography increased between 1980 and 1985 in the elderly, and then declined (fig. 6).[21,22] Rates of both procedures were much lower in elderly Blacks than would be

Table III. Number of first-listed diagnoses of cerebrovascular disease, days of care and all-listed cerebrovascular procedures: US, 1993 (from National Hospital Discharge Survey[19,20])

	First-listed diagnoses		Days of care		All-listed procedures	
	no. (thousands)	rate (per 100 000)	no. (thousands)	rate (per 100 000)	no. (thousands)	rate (per 100 000)
Cerebrovascular disease	841	328	7080	2761		
intracranial haemorrhage[a]	61	24	642	250		
thromboembolic stroke[b]	274	107	2651	1034		
ill-defined stroke[c]	169	66	1675	653		
Carotid endarterectomy					63	35
Carotid arteriography					45	37

a ICD9-CM 431-432.
b ICD9-CM 434.
c ICD9-CM 436.
no. = number of diagnoses, days or procedures.

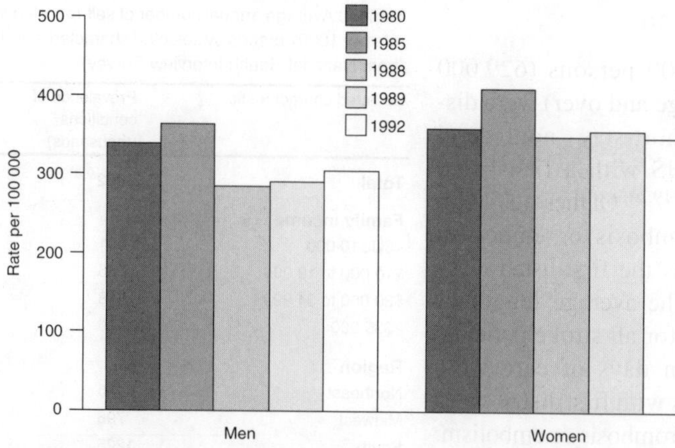

Fig. 3. Rate of hospital discharge in the US (1980 to 1992) with a first-listed diagnosis of cerebrovascular disease by sex (from National Hospital Discharge Survey[19,20]).

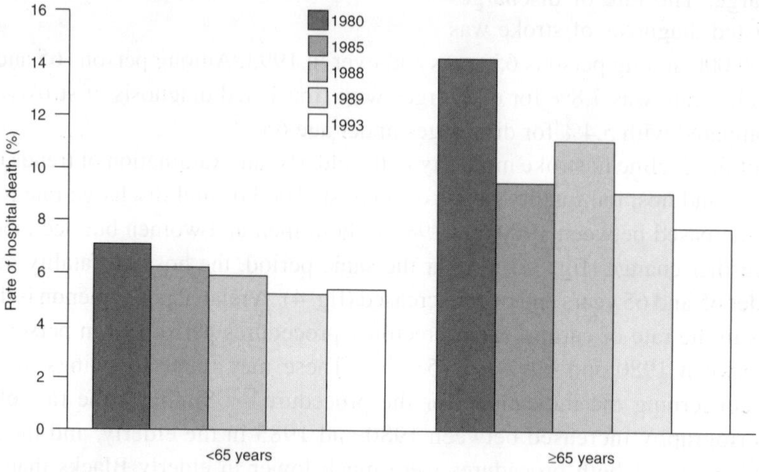

Fig. 4. Rate of hospital death among discharges in the US (1980 to 1993) with a first-listed diagnosis of cerebrovascular disease by age (from National Hospital Discharge Survey[19,20]).

expected based on stroke mortality rates.[22] Thus, the only important change in outcomes and utilisation of hospital services for stroke to accompany declining mortality in the elderly was declining hospital case fatality.

2.3 Ambulatory Care

In the 1994 National Ambulatory Medical Care Survey, there were 2.096 million visits to office-based physicians with principal diagnosis of stroke, 1.592 million in persons 65 years and over.[23-25] Of these, 57% were visits to internists or general practitioners, and 16% were to neurologists.[26] Of the 2 million total visits, 72% were visits involving drug therapy. In 18% of persons visiting physicians for stroke, four or more drugs were ordered or provided at the stroke visit.

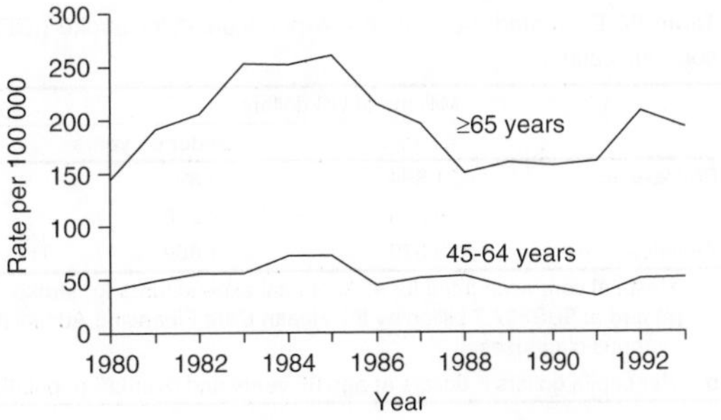

Fig. 5. Rate of all-listed carotid endarterectomy in the US (1980 to 1993) by age (from Gillum,[22] with permission).

2.4 Nursing Home Care

In the National Nursing Home Survey of 1985, cerebrovascular disease accounted for about 12% of all primary admission diagnoses and about 11% of diagnoses at discharge.[27] Of 142 600 discharged patients admitted with a primary diagnosis of stroke, 67.3% were discharged alive. Average duration of stay was 348 days, median duration was 82 days; 31.6% stayed 6 months or more. The median age was 81 years, with 32.7% aged 85 or over and 93.1% aged 65 or over. Women comprised 62.1%. Prior to nursing home admission, 63.2% were in a short-stay hospital. Among persons aged 65 years and over in nursing homes, the prevalence of stroke was 193.3 per 1000 compared with 59.3 among community dwelling elderly.[28] Nursing home residents with stroke had an average of 4.5 dependencies compared with 3.8 for all residents.

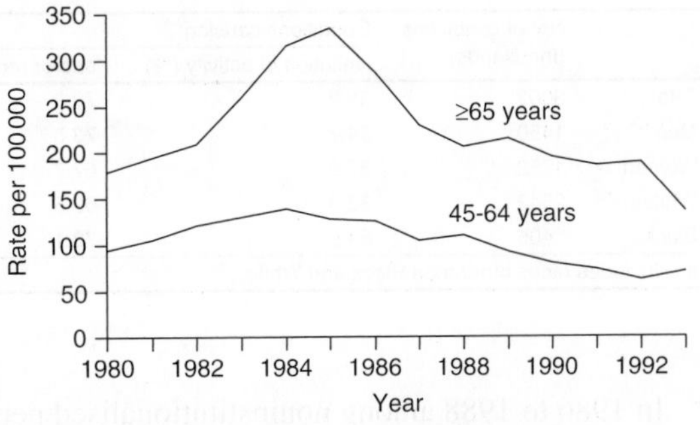

Fig. 6. Rate of all-listed cerebral arteriography in the US (1980 to 1993) by age (from Gillum,[22] with permission).

2.5 The Last Year of Life

Data from the 1986 National Mortality Follow-back Survey revealed that a somewhat larger proportion of persons dying of stroke (30% of women, 10% of men) had resided in an institution in the preceding year compared with persons dying of other causes.[4] Among stroke decedents, 27% had 1 to 4 doctor visits and 35% had 5 to 14 doctor visits in the preceding year.[4] The proportion receiving assistance in activities of daily living (45%) was similar in persons dying of stroke compared with other causes.

2.6 Healthcare Expenditures and Disability

Recent cost figures for stroke are shown in table IV. Nearly 18 thousand million US dollars were spent for stroke care in 1995 in the US (Thomas A. Hodgson, personal communication). Clearly this entity is a major contributor to the total expenditures for cardiovascular disease.[29,30] Hospital care accounted for 42% of the totals.

Table IV. Estimated medical care expenditures[a] for stroke (ICD9-CM 430-438) in the US, 1995 (T.A. Hodgson, personal communication)

	Millions of US dollars			Per capita (US dollars)[b]
	All ages	Under 65 years	65 years and over	65 years and over
Both sexes	21 894	3 895	17 999	537
Males	8 215	2 226	5 989	438
Females	13 679	1 669	12 010	605

a Hospital care accounted for 42% of total expenditures for stroke. Total personal medical care expenditures in 1995 were estimated at $US897.7 billion by the Health Care Financing Administration. Of this total it is possible to allocate about 88% to various diagnoses.

b Per capita dollars = dollars at age 65 years and over/US population 65 years and over.

Table V. Average annual number of self-reported chronic stroke conditions among persons by sex and race, and percentage of conditions causing activity limitation, hospitalisation and physician visits: US, 1990 to 1992 (from National Health Interview Survey)

	No. of conditions (thousands)	Conditions causing:		
		limitation of activity (%)	one or more hospitalisations (%)	one or more physician visits (%)
Total[a]	3002	35.9	70.3	99.6
Men	1450	34.7	73.0	99.1
Women	1552	37.0	67.7	100.0
Whites	2549	33.3	69.5	99.5
Blacks	405	54.6	73.1	100.0

a Includes races other than Black and White.

In 1986 to 1988 among noninstitutionalised persons, 42.9% of men and 36.0% of women, 36.6% of Whites and 55.3% of Blacks with self-reported stroke had activity limitation.[31] Rates of disability were similar in 1990 to 1992 (table V). Also shown are percentages of prevalent cases reporting hospital and physician utilisation in the preceding year. Rates of disability among elderly persons with stroke were quite high and increased with age.[31] At age 75 years and over, 76% of men and 55% of women with stroke were restricted in their usual activity.[31] Further, disability rates in men aged from 60 to 69 years increased between 1969 and 1980.[32]

3. Conclusions

This article has summarised data from the National Center for Health Statistics on the burden of stroke in the US population with particular attention to those aged 65 years and over. Despite downward trends, stroke remains the third leading cause of death. Further, stroke is the cause of morbidity and utilisation of health services and disability in increasing numbers of persons over the age of 65 years.

With respect to patterns of occurrence of stroke by age and sex in the elderly, data from the National Center for Health Statistics are generally consistent with data from other epidemiological studies of stroke.[33-35] Data are inadequate on the epidemiology of stroke in Blacks and other racial minorities.[12,36,37] Limitations of the data presented have been discussed in detail elsewhere.[1,2,4-6,8-16,18-31,35-38] However, these are not likely to affect the broad conclusions summarised above. Increasing or stable national hospitalisation rates for stroke are somewhat surprising because of several studies showing decreasing incidence of stroke in young and old in the 1950s to 1970s and declining mortality in the 1980s.[33,34]

Controversy has arisen as to whether incidence has failed to decrease or actually increased since then.[33,34,39,40] This suggests that the decrease in case fatality of acute stroke and increase in survivorship following stroke may have lead to rising stroke prevalence especially in the elderly.[35,41] In combination with the increase in the population aged 65 years and over, this has lead to recent increases in the utilisation of hospital, ambulatory and chronic care services for stroke in the elderly.[42,43] These increases are likely to continue unless the incidence of stroke can be drastically reduced. This stresses the need for even more vigorous efforts at primary prevention of stroke to reduce the burden of illness and not just the mortality rate from stroke.[44]

Key points:

- In 1993, 150 108 deaths were attributed to stroke, the third leading cause of death.
- Death rates were lower in Whites than in Blacks with the exception of ages 85 and over.
- There were probably nearly 3 million persons with diagnosed stroke in the civilian non-institutionalised population in the US in 1994.
- In 1993, over 841 000 persons were discharged from short-stay hospitals with a principal diagnosis of stroke.
- The hospital fatality rate was 7.8% for all cerebrovascular disease.
- Since 1988, hospitalisation rates for stroke have changed little while hospital fatality rates have decreased.
- Nearly 18 thousand million US dollars were spent for stroke care in 1995 in the US.
- More vigorous efforts at primary prevention of stroke are needed to reduce the burden of illness and restore the decline in mortality rate from stroke.

Future research needs to include:

- Further studies of the validity of stroke mortality and morbidity rates, especially in Blacks and other minorities.
- Studies of the correlates of geographic variation in stroke mortality and morbidity.
- Studies of trends in mortality, incidence, survivorship, prevalence and medical care of stroke in the White and Black population to determine the cause of the deceleration and possible reversal of the long term decline in mortality.
- Studies of the utilisation of carotid endarterectomy surgery and carotid arteriography in White and Black persons with cerebrovascular disease.

Acknowledgements

We wish to thank the staff of the National Center for Health Statistics of the Centers for Disease Control and Prevention. Special thanks are due to David Woodwell for providing data on ambulatory care of stroke, to Thomas A. Hodgson, PhD for providing data on the costs of stroke, and to John Gary Collins for providing unpublished data on stroke prevalence and disability.

References

1. National Center for Health Statistics. Advance report of final mortality statistics, 1993. Monthly vital statistics report. Hyattsville (MD): Public Health Service, 1996 Feb 29; 44 (7) Suppl. DHHS Pub. no. (PHS) 96-1120
2. National Center for Health Statistics. Vital Statistics of the United States, 1990. Vol. II, Mortality, part A. Public Health Service. Washington, DC: US Government Printing Office, 1994. DHHS Pub. no. (PHS) 95-1101
3. World Health Organization. Manual of the international statistical classification of diseases, injuries, and causes of death, based on the recommendations of the Ninth Revision Conference, 1975. Geneva: World Health Organization, 1977

4. National Center for Health Statistics, Powell-Griner E. Characteristics of persons dying from cerebrovascular diseases: preliminary data from the 1986 National Mortality Followback Survey. In: Advance data from vital and health statistics: no.s 171-180. Vital and health statistics. Hyattsville (MD): Public Health Service, 1995; 16 (18). PHS Pub. no. 95-1877
5. National Center for Health Statistics. The National Health Interview Survey design, 1973-84, and procedures, 1975-83. National Center for Health Statistics. Vital Health Stat 1 1985; 18
6. National Center for Health Statistics, Simmons WR. Development of the design of the NCHS Hospital Discharge Survey. Vital and health statistics. Public Health Service. Washington, DC: Public Health Service, 1970 Sep; 2 (39). PHS Pub. no. 1000
7. The international classification of diseases, 9th revision, clinical modification. Public Health Service. 3rd ed. Washington, DC: US Government Printing Office, 1989. DHHS Pub. no. (PHS) 89-1260
8. National Center for Health Statistics. Bryant E, Shimizu I. Sample design, sampling variance, and estimation procedures for the National Ambulatory Medical Care Survey. National Center for Health Statistics. Vital Health Stat 1988; 2 (108)
9. National Center for Health Statistics. Ingram DK. Profile of chronic illness in nursing homes, United States, National Nursing Home Survey, August 1973-April 1974. National Center for Health Statistics. Vital Health Stat 1977; 13 (29)
10. National Center for Health Statistics, Kovar MG. Data systems of the National Center for Health Statistics. Vital and health statistics. Hyattsville (MD): Public Health Service, 1989 Mar; 1 (23). DHHS Pub. no. (PHS) 89-1325
11. National Center for Health Statistics. Multiple causes of death in the United States. Monthly vital statistics report. Hyattsville (MD): Public Health Service, 1984 Feb 17; 32 (10 Suppl. 2). PHHS Pub. no. (PHS) 84-1120
12. Gillum RF. The epidemiology of stroke in Hispanics in the United States. Stroke 1995; 26: 1707-12
13. National Center for Health Statistics, Pickle L, Mungiole M. Atlas of mortality United States, 1988-92. Hyattsville (MD): Public Health Service, 1997. DHHS Pub. no. (PHS) 97-1015
14. National Center for Health Statistics, Cohen BB, Kleinman JC. Death rates from ischemic heart and other related diseases by health service area, 1968-72. Statistical notes for health planners no. 10. Hyattsville (MD): Public Health Service, 1979. DHEW Pub. no. (PHS) 80-1237
15. Gillum RF, Ingram DI. The relation between residence in the Southeast region of the United States and stroke incidence and death: the NHANES I Epidemiologic follow-Up Study. Am J Epidemiol 1996; 144: 665-73
16. Zarate AO. International mortality chart book. Levels and trends, 1955-91. Hyattsville (MD): Public Health Service, 1994
17. Gillum RF, Feinleib M. Cardiovascular disease in the United States: mortality, prevalence, and incidence. In: Kapoor AS, Singh BN, editors. Prognosis and risk assessment in cardiovascular disease. New York: Churchill Livingstone Inc., 1993: 49-59
18. National Center for Health Statistics. Prevalence of selected chronic circulatory conditions United States 1986-88. Vital and health statistics. Hyattsville (MD): Public Health Service, 1993 Feb; 10 (182). DHHS Pub. no. (PHS) 93-1510
19. National Center for Health Statistics, Graves, EJ. National Hospital Discharge Survey: annual summary, 1993. Vital and health statistics. Washington, DC: Public Health Service, 1995 Aug; 13 (121). DHHS Pub. no. (PHS) 95-1782
20. National Center for Health Statistics, Graves EJ. Detailed diagnoses and procedures, National Hospital Discharge Survey, 1993. Vital and health statistics. Washington, DC: Public Health Service, 1995 Oct; 13 (122). DHHS Pub. no. (PHS) 95-1783
21. Gillum RF. Cerebrovascular disease morbidity in the United States, 1974-1983: age, sex, race region and vascular surgery. Stroke 1986; 17: 656-61
22. Gillum RF. Epidemiology of carotid endarterectomy and cerebral arteriography in the United States. Stroke 1995; 26: 1724-8
23. National Center for Health Statistics, Cypress BK. Office visits for diseases of the circulatory system. The National Ambulatory Medical Care Survey United States, 1975-1976. Vital and health statistics. Hyattsville (MD): Public Health Service, 1979 Jan; 13 (40). DHEW Pub. no. (PHS) 79-1791
24. National Center for Health Statistics, Hing E, Cypress BK. Use of health services by women 65 years of age and over United States. Vital and health statistics. Hyattsville (MD): Public Health Service, 1981 Aug; 13 (59). DHHS Pub. no. (PHS) 81-1720
25. National Center for Health Statistics, Schappert SM. National Ambulatory Medical Care Survey: 1989 Summary. National Center for Health Statistics. Vital Health Stat 1992; 13 (110)
26. National Center for Health Statistics, Nelson C, McLemore T. The National Ambulatory Medical Care Survey, United States, 1975-81 and 1985 trends. National Center for Health Statistics. Vital Health Stat 1988; 13 (93)
27. National Center for Health Statistics, Sekscenski ES. Discharges from nursing homes: 1985 National Nursing Home Survey. Vital and health statistics. Hyattsville (MD): Public Health Service, 1990 Mar; 13 (103). DHHS Pub. no. (PHS) 90-1764
28. National Center for Health Statistics, Hing E. Nursing home utilization by current residents: United States, 1985. Vital and health statistics. Hyattsville (MD): Public Health Service, 1989 Oct; 13 (102). DHHS Pub. no. (PHS) 89-1763
29. Hodgson TA, Kopstein AN. Health Care expenditures for major diseases in 1980. Health Care Financ Rev 1984; 5: 1-12
30. Hodgson TA. Health care expenditures for major diseases in 1980. Health Care Financ Rev 1984; 6: 128-30
31. National Center for Health Statistics, Collins JG. Prevalence of selected chronic conditions: United States 1986-88. Vital and health statistics. Hyattsville (MD): Public Health Service, 1993 Feb; 10 (182). DHHS Pub. no. (PHS) 93-1510
32. Feldman JJ. Work ability of the aged under conditions of improving mortality. Milbank Mem Fund Q 1983; 61: 430-44
33. Whisnant JP, editor. Stroke: populations, cohorts, and clinical trials. Oxford: Butterworth-Heineman Ltd., 1993
34. Klag MJ, Whelton PK. The decline in stroke mortality: an epidemiologic perspective. Ann Epidemiol 1993; 3: 571-5
35. Thom TJ. Stroke mortality trends: an international perspective. Ann Epidemiol 1993; 3: 509-18
36. Gillum RF. The epidemiology of stroke in Native Americans. Stroke 1995; 26: 514-21

37. Gillum RF: Stroke in blacks. Stroke 1988; 19: 1-9
38. National Center for Health Statistics: Health United States 1995. Hyattsville (MD): Public Health Service, 1996 May: 129-31. DHHS Pub. no. (PHS) 96-1232
39. Broderick JP, Phillips SJ, Whisnant JP, et al. Incidence rates of stroke in the eighties: the end of the decline in stroke? Stroke 1989; 20: 577-82
40. Brown Jr RD, Whisnant JP, Sicks JD, et al. Stroke incidence, prevalence, and survival: secular trends in Rochester, Minnesota, through 1989. Stroke 1996; 27: 373-80
41. Kovar MG, Pokras R, Collins JG. Trends in medical care and survival from stroke. Ann Epidemiol 1993; 3: 466-70
42. Rice DP, Feldman JJ. Living longer in the United States: demographic changes and health needs of the elderly. Milbank Mem Fund Q 1983; 61: 362-96
43. Manton KG, Soldo BJ. Dynamics of health changes in the oldest old: new perspectives and evidence. Milbank Mem Fund Q 1985; 63: 206-85
44. Healthy people 2000: national health promotion and disease prevention objectives (1991). Washington, DC: US Department of Health and Human Services, Public Health Service, 1991. DHHS Publication no. PHS 91-50212

Correspondence: Dr *Richard F. Gillum,* Centers for Disease Control and Prevention, Office of Analysis, Epidemiology and Health Promotion, National Center for Health Statistics, 6525 Belcrest Road, Hyattsville, MD 20782, USA.

Cost Considerations in the Pharmacological Prevention and Treatment of Stroke

Andrei V. Alexandrov, Liliana T. Smurawska, William Bartle and *Paul Oh*

Stroke Research Unit and the Division of Clinical Pharmacology, Sunnybrook Health Science Centre, University of Toronto, Toronto, Ontario, Canada

Stroke constitutes one of the most frequent causes of morbidity and mortality in North America and worldwide. The American Heart Association (AHA) released the 1992 Heart and Stroke Facts[1] in which the incidence of stroke in the US was estimated at 400 000 to 500 000 new cases per year, with an estimated prevalence of 3 million stroke survivors.

Stroke is a common cause of hospital admissions in the US, accounting for almost 1% of all such admissions nationwide.[2] Approximately 150 000 deaths are attributed to stroke, making it the third leading cause of mortality after cancer and heart disease, according to the 1991 Advance Report on Final Mortality Statistics in the US.[1] AHA Stroke Facts[1] reports that about 140 000 individuals in the US are transferred to nursing homes each year following a nonfatal stroke, while the total estimated cost for stroke care for both direct healthcare expenditures and indirect economic losses is about $US30 billion per year.

With recent debate over potential cost savings on healthcare and particularly on limiting aggressiveness of care in terminally ill patients,[3] cost considerations implied by stroke prevention and treatment strategies should not be left unattended.

Age-adjusted stroke mortality rates have been decreasing for the last few decades, mainly because of reductions in stroke severity and mortality in patients under 70 years of age; there have also been reductions in the incidence of intracerebral haemorrhages, as a result of continuing improvement in the control of hypertension.[4-8] However, since the population as a whole has aged, the overall incidence of stroke has not followed a clear pattern of decline,[8] and thus the costs for stroke care may rise further in the future.

The goal of this review is to summarise current knowledge on the effectiveness and costs of the most widely used therapies for acute stroke and its secondary prevention.

There are several areas in which pharmacological therapy might have an impact on the incidence and the economic ramifications of stroke, and we will examine these in turn under the categories of prevention strategies and acute stroke treatments.

1. Stroke Prevention and Major Risk Factors

The major modifiable risk factors for stroke were recently summarised by Gorelick,[6] and include hypertension, cigarette smoking, atrial fibrillation and heavy alcohol consumption.

Table I. Modifiable risk factors, population-attributable risk and potential number of strokes that could be prevented by elimination of each factor in the US (data modified from Gorelick[6]). The potential number of strokes prevented was calculated on the basis of 500 000 new strokes annually

Risk factor	Population-attributable risk (%)	Potential number of strokes prevented
Hypertension	49.3	246 500
Smoking	12.3	61 500
Atrial fibrillation	9.4	47 000
Heavy alcohol consumption	4.7	23 500

Table I shows the population-attributable risks along with the projected number of strokes that might be prevented by means of elimination of these factors. Hypertension was the single strongest risk factor for the population in this and other reviews.[6-8] Aggressive identification and management of hypertension, such as through the National High Blood Pressure Education Programme in the US, has resulted in a decline in the incidence of intracerebral haemorrhage and stroke mortality rates,[7,8] allowing some reviewers to suggest that up to 70% of strokes could be eliminated by the treatment of hypertension alone.[4-6]

Mortality from stroke (according to the registry at Rochester, Minnesota, US) declined from 33% in 1949 to 17% by 1984, mainly as a result of reductions in mortality in patients less than 70 years old and in the incidence of intracerebral haemorrhage.[7] In the Framingham study,[8] the reduction in stroke mortality resulted from a significant decline in stroke severity, but not stroke incidence; notably, the incidence of isolated transient ischaemic attacks (TIAs) was higher in this study compared with previous reports.[8] Recent developments in diagnostic strategies have formed the basis for better recognition of stroke and its pathogenic mechanisms. Improvements in computed tomography, cerebral angiography and, most recently, cardiovascular ultrasound have also identified more individuals who are suitable for treatment by means of early recognition of a high-risk profile for subsequent stroke.[7-10]

The ability of antihypertensive drug therapy to reduce the risk of stroke has been unequivocally demonstrated in a number of clinical trials. The large meta-analysis reported by Collins et al.[11] in 1990 showed that there was a 42% reduction in the rate of stroke with antihypertensive therapy. It should be noted that the main therapies studied thus far in these trials have been diuretics and β-blockers.

Economic appraisals of antihypertensive therapy for the prevention of stroke have suggested that blood pressure reduction is indeed a cost-effective strategy, with an incremental cost per quality-adjusted life year (QALY) gained in the order of $US10 000 to $US20 000 per year.[12,13] However, some of these data have come into question, since more recent economic appraisals have suggested lower net benefits of blood pressure treatment than previously projected;[4,14] and incremental cost-effectiveness ratios have become less favourable, ranging from 11 058 to 63 760 pounds sterling (£) [equivalent to approximately $US17 400 to $US100 000] per QALY gained in a study from New Zealand.[4] In all of these analyses, the conclusions were sensitive to the type of therapy employed, with diuretics consistently being the most attractive in terms of net benefits and cost effectiveness, and the patient risk profiles influencing the potential gains over time.

Gorelick[6] went on further and tried to extrapolate the savings that could be realised through the modification of risk factors; these savings are shown in table II. At various levels of risk-factor control in stroke prevention, potential savings in direct and indirect costs could be seen. For instance, if hypertension could be eliminated completely, there might be annual economic savings of $US12.33 billion, most of which can be attributed to the costs of acute treatment.

There is an opportunity to intervene with pharmacological agents that aid smoking cessation, but given that these are relatively new therapies, long term data in terms of outcome prevention have not yet been reported and thus long term economic evaluations are unavailable.

Table II. Projected cost savings (1991 values) through stroke prevention (data modified from Gorelick[6])

Cost savings by risk factor	Level of success in preventing stroke		
	100%	50%	10%
Total annual economic savings ($US billions)[a]			
Hypertension	12.33	6.17	1.23
Smoking	3.08	1.54	0.31
Economic savings for acute hospital stay ($US billions)[b]			
Hypertension	11.33	5.67	1.13
Smoking	2.83	1.42	0.28

a Calculations are based on $US25 billion spent per year in stroke care; 100% values refer to the prevention of 246 500 strokes among patients with hypertension and 61 500 strokes among smokers.

b Calculations are based on $US46 000 per patient with acute stroke in a Chicago hospital in 1991.

2. Stroke Prevention Therapy

2.1 Antiplatelet Agents

Aspirin (acetylsalicylic acid) is the least expensive and most widely available drug used in stroke prevention (table III).[15] The benefits of aspirin in preventing stroke were first reported in 1956 by Dr L.L. Craven, a family physician from Glendale, California, US. Since then a number of large prospective randomised trials have been conducted, with the cumulative evidence suggesting that aspirin reduces the incidence of nonfatal ischaemic stroke by 22%, and the constellation of nonfatal stroke, myocardial infarction or vascular death by 25% (relative risk reduction) compared with placebo.[16] Complications, primarily gastrointestinal (GI) and intracerebral bleeding, have been reported with long term therapy and may be dosage-related.[15-17] However, because the magnitude of the benefits is high relative to the low cost of therapy, aspirin is a cost-saving intervention in the prevention of stroke.[15-17]

As an antiplatelet agent, aspirin is the mainstay of preventive antithrombotic therapy for primary cerebrovascular disease.[17] When patients cannot tolerate aspirin because of adverse effects (e.g GI bleeding) or present with failure of aspirin therapy (e.g. stroke or TIA), they are usually prescribed ticlopidine. In patients who had experienced a recent TIA, reversible ischaemic neurological deficit, amaurosis fugax or minor stroke, ticlopidine reduced the incidence of new strokes by 21%, compared with aspirin.[15-17] However, in the meta-analysis published by the Anti-Platelet Trialists' Collaborative Group,[18] there was no statistically significant difference in outcome in favour of ticlopidine; although the point estimate showed a 10% odds reduction with ticlopidine, the 95% confidence intervals overlapped with an odds ratio of 1.[18] Treatment with ticlopidine is associated with higher daily acquisition costs and incidence of some adverse effects, such as neutropenia, and thus its use may be limited.[17,19]

To analyse the effect of the higher costs and improved outcomes with ticlopidine, Oster and colleagues[20] performed a cost-effectiveness analysis using decision-analytic modelling. In a simulated cohort of 100 high-risk men and women who were at least 65 years of age and received either ticlopidine 250mg per day or aspirin 1300 mg/day, 2 fewer strokes occurred in the ticlopidine group over the life expectancy of the cohort. The increased acquisition cost of therapy in the ticlopidine group ($US2939 per patient compared to $US135 per patient in the aspirin group, discounted over 5 years (5% per year; initial costing 1991) was somewhat offset by the lower lifetime costs of stroke-specific care with ticlopidine ($US8539 and $US9219, respectively). The overall lifetime medical-care costs, including treatment for GI haemorrhage

Table III. Pharmacological agents used to prevent ischaemic stroke, and their associated costs

Agent	Use	Dosage	Acquisition cost per day ($US)	NNT	Major complication	Cost per complication ($US)
Aspirin (acetylsalicylic acid)	Primary/secondary prevention	325 (range 30-1300) mg/day	0.13	167	GI bleeding 2.48% (1.7% hospitalised)[20]	48-4997[a]
	Nonvalvular atrial fibrillation	325 mg/day		83		
Ticlopidine	Secondary prevention	250 mg/day	2.75	28	Neutropenia 2.3%[19]b	96-8028[a]
Warfarin	Primary/secondary prevention, nonvalvular atrial fibrillation	Titrated to achieve INR 2-3 (limits 1.5-4)	0.18[c]	28	ICH 1.3%[23]d	0-9000[e]

a Medicare charges in 1991.[15]

b Ticlopidine Aspirin Stroke Study Group data.[19]

c Cost of warfarin is given for a 5mg tablet, Ontario Drug Benefit Formulary, 1995.

d 20% fatal, 11% mild-to-severe, 69% no residual.[23]

e Diagnosis related group 14, 1994.[25]

GI = gastrointestinal; **ICH** = intracerebral haemorrhage; **INR** = international normalised ratio; **NNT** = number needed to treat to prevent 1 stroke per year.

and neutropenia, were $US2341 higher in the ticlopidine group ($US64 443 *vs* $US62 102). The benefits of ticlopidine were also expressed as a gain in quality-adjusted life expectancy that ranged from 0.04 to 0.07 years, thus yielding a mean incremental cost per QALY gained of $US39 900. The use of ticlopidine is therefore moderately cost effective compared with aspirin in the secondary prevention of stroke.

Although the debate over the relative benefits of ticlopidine and aspirin continues,[21-23] aspirin should not be viewed as a harmless drug, since it is associated with a relatively high (dosage-related) incidence of GI bleeding (2.48%)[24] and intracerebral bleeding (0.3%).[23]

The cost effectiveness of ticlopidine is likely to be country-dependent.[23] For instance, stroke-related direct healthcare costs are greater in Canada than in the USA because of the open-ended nature of the government-funded healthcare system, resulting in a greater length of in-hospital stay for patients with an acute stroke.[25] Thus, the prevention of just two more strokes per 100 patients using ticlopidine would result in greater cost savings in a setting with a healthcare system similar to that of Canada.

For the individual patient, the factors that should be considered in choosing an antiplatelet agent should include: past neurological history (e.g. cerebrovascular events); intolerance to, or failure of, aspirin therapy; expected compliance with haematological monitoring; and, perhaps, ability to pay the higher drug acquisition cost.[17,19,23]

2.2 Anticoagulants

2.2.1 Indications

Determination of one of the three main pathogenic mechanisms of ischaemic stroke, i.e. cardioembolic, atherothrombotic or lacunar, is of paramount importance in determining further pharmacological intervention in the individual patient. Other mechanisms and aetiologies, such as arterial dissection, patent foramen ovale, sickle cell disease and coagulopathies, are less common and require separate consideration, particularly in patients with strokes that remain 'cryptogenic' after initial diagnostic work-up or in a young patient.

Brain cardioembolism often occurs in patients with nonvalvular atrial fibrillation (NVAF), a condition that affects approximately 2 million people in the US.[26] Cumulative data suggest that individuals with atrial fibrillation (of all types) have a 3.6-fold greater relative risk of sustaining a stroke than those with normal sinus rhythm, resulting in a stroke risk of approximately 5% per year.[7,26,27]

Eight recently completed randomised clinical trials have focused on prevention of strokes in patients with NVAF.[27-33] The effectiveness of warfarin therapy was documented, and in three trials, warfarin was compared with aspirin and placebo.[27,30,31] Aspirin itself was effective in only one of these trials,[27] but because of the increased risk of haemorrhage in warfarin-treated patients, there is a renewed interest in treating low-risk patients with aspirin.[16,29]

2.2.2 Warfarin versus Aspirin

Level of Stroke Risk

Gage and colleagues[29] used a Markov decision-analytic model to compare aspirin with warfarin in patients with NVAF. They divided the population into 3 groups, based on the presence or absence of additional risk factors (i.e. a history of stroke or TIA, diabetes, hypertension or heart disease): high stroke risk with multiple risk factors (5.3% per year), medium risk with one additional risk factor (3.6% per year), and low risk with only NVAF (1.6% per year). Aspirin therapy was assumed to be associated with a 22% relative reduction in risk of stroke, warfarin therapy with a relative risk reduction of 68%. The annual rate of haemorrhage with warfarin was assumed to be 1.4%.

In the high-risk population, the quality-adjusted life expectancy over 10 years of analysis for a cohort of patients who were 65 years old was 6.51 years for warfarin, 6.27 years with aspirin and 6.01 years with no therapy. Overall, warfarin was the least expensive therapy ($US12 500 compared with $US13 200 for aspirin and $US15 300 for no therapy; 1994 costs) as a result of savings in stroke-management costs that were more than enough to offset the additional costs associated with drug monitoring and adverse events with warfarin. In the medium-risk population, aspirin was the least expensive therapy at $US9700, compared with $US10 900 for warfarin. The warfarin strategy was associated with a gain of 0.14 QALYs and thus an incremental ratio of $US8000 per QALY gained, compared with aspirin. In those patients with a very low risk of stroke, aspirin again was the least expensive therapy and the expected number of QALYs for warfarin and aspirin was virtually the same at 6.70 and 6.69, respectively.

Thus, in high-risk individuals, warfarin would be the preferred therapy, whereas in low-risk individuals, aspirin would seem to be the most prudent choice. In those with an intermediate risk, the incremental ratio for warfarin was quite attractive, but therapeutic decisions should be individualised according to patient stroke risk factors and preference. Ongoing randomised trials will provide further information on the effectiveness of aspirin in this group of patients to help in the decision-making process.

Risk of Adverse Effects

Gustafsson et al.,[33] projected the cost effectiveness of anticoagulant and antiplatelet therapy for atrial fibrillation for the entire Swedish population. The authors estimated that there were 83 000 individuals in Sweden who had atrial fibrillation, of whom 22 000 would be potential candidates for anticoagulants and 55 000 for aspirin. The estimated annual cost of stroke therapy per patient in Swedish krona (SEK) was SEK180 000 in direct costs and SEK90 000 in indirect costs (SEK100 = $US15; costs and exchange rate estimates from 1991). The baseline annual stroke rate was 5% per year and the relative stroke reduction that might be achieved with anticoagulants and aspirin was estimated at 64% and 25%, respectively. The risk of intracranial haemorrhage with warfarin was set at 3 levels, 0.3, 1.3 and 2.0% per year.

The estimated annual cost of treatment was SEK5030 for anticoagulants and SEK100 for aspirin. Without specific therapy, 3850 ischaemic strokes would be expected in the eligible cohort of approximately 75 000 individuals. Using warfarin in the appropriate patients would have the largest net benefit in terms of stroke reduction by preventing 410 events, assuming an intermediate risk of haemorrhage (1.3%). The additional use of aspirin in the remaining 55 000 individuals would prevent a further 670 strokes. This translates into an annual rate of stroke reduction of 127 per million inhabitants in Sweden, with a net saving of SEK21 million ($US3.15 million). The study authors[33] concluded that treatment with anticoagulants or, if warfarin was contraindicated, with aspirin was the most cost-effective strategy, provided that the risk of serious haemorrhagic complications was kept low.

3. Acute Stroke Treatment

3.1 Heparin

In addition to prevention, anticoagulation is also employed in the acute treatment of patients with cerebral ischaemia. Heparin, an agent that prevents conversion of prothrombin to thrombin, has been tested in a number of clinical trials. However, the effectiveness of heparin in reducing disability and stroke recurrence remains controversial.[34] Therefore, current neurological practice is to reserve the use of heparin for those individuals who have cardioembolic stroke, acute partial stable stroke or show progression or fluctuation of the initial neurological deficit and who have no evidence of large volume ischaemic lesions on computed tomography (CT) scan. Heparin is also used in patients with crescendo TIAs and signs of basilar artery thrombosis.[34-36] However, formulation of evidence-based guidelines must await publication of the results of the International Stroke Trial.[37]

One of the most serious complications of heparin is thought to be haemorrhagic conversion of a brain infarction. The Cerebral Embolism Study Group[38] reported that haemorrhagic transformation of infarctions that were initially pale on CT scanning occurred after 48 hours in 5% of all patients with embolic stroke and in 18% of those with large infarctions. However, the study size was too small to draw definite conclusions on the risk of bleeding with intravenous heparin. In another study,[39] 3058 patients with acute stroke were screened, but only 225 were given heparin. No stroke progression as a result of bleeding complications was reported in the heparin group, presumably because of rigid inclusion criteria, which probably improved the tolerability of anticoagulation therapy, but limited its applicability.[39] Since the first clinical trials did not show sufficient evidence of benefits from heparin,[38,39] cost-effectiveness studies are not available.

3.2 Low-Molecular-Weight Heparins

In the past few years, trials have been conducted with the new generation of anticoagulants, the low–molecular-weight (LMW) heparins.

Table IV. Pharmacological agents for treatment of acute ischaemic stroke and costs (1996 values). Costs of complications remain to be determined for all 3 agents

Agent	Time window	Dosage	Acquisition cost per day ($US)	No. needed to treat[a]	Major complication
Heparin	First 48 hours	Adjusted to APTT[b]	5	Not known	Intracerebral haemorrhage (rate 1%[37])
Nadroparin	First 48 hours	4100IU twice daily subcutaneously	8-20[c]	5	Intracerebral haemorrhage (rate not known)
Alteplase	First 3 hours	Up to 90mg intravenously (bolus 10%; infusion 90% over 1h)	1640	8	Intracerebral haemorrhage (6.4%)[46]

a Number of patients needed to treat in order to reverse 1 stroke or prevent 1 death. Outcome data to estimate number needed to treat for nadroparin and alteplase.[40,46]

b The activated partial thromboplastin time (APTT) is kept at 50 to 70 seconds, or at 1.5 to 2.5 times the pretreatment level.

c Estimated from the costs of other low–molecular-weight heparins, tinzaparin and enoxaparin, which are currently available in Canada.

A recent trial of nadroparin was reported by Kay et al.[40] In this multicentre study conducted in Hong Kong, nadroparin (4100 anti-factor Xa IU subcutaneously twice daily for 10 days) was shown to be superior to placebo if it was administered within 48 hours of an acute ischaemic stroke. The data suggested that for every 5 patients treated, 1 death or case of severe disability was avoided. These results are quite encouraging, but need to be explored in further prospective studies.

It is possible that the Chinese population studied in the trial of Kay et al.[40] benefited to a greater extent because of the higher prevalence of intracranial arterial stenoses in this population;[41] the results may not be similar in western populations. A formal economic evaluation has not yet been performed on this trial,[40] but preliminary analysis by our group suggests that the relatively small drug expenditures associated with LMW heparins [approximately 100 Canadian dollars ($Can) per 10-day course in Ontario, Canada] and the possible large gain (up to 20% absolute risk reduction in death or dependency), makes nadroparin a very attractive intervention ($US1.00 ≈ $Can1.30). Further multinational trials of nadroparin are needed to more precisely determine the efficacy and cost effectiveness of this agent in patients with acute ischaemic stroke.

3.3 Thrombolytics

Another aspect of early intervention in acute ischaemic stroke follows the major new intervention in coronary artery disease over the last decade, i.e. intravenous thrombolysis. Thrombolytic agents administered during the so-called 'therapeutic window' in patients with an acute stroke have, to date, been tested in five major international randomised trials.[42-46] Three trials evaluated streptokinase administered within 4 and 6 hours after stroke onset and were all terminated because of excessive numbers of deaths and haemorrhagic complications in the treatment groups, compared with placebo.[42-44] The other 2 trials evaluated alteplase (recombinant tissue plasminogen activator; r-tPA) [table IV].[45,46]

3.3.1 Studies with Alteplase

The European Cooperative Acute Stroke Study (ECASS) found no benefit of thrombolysis, as a result of the high rate of haemorrhagic conversion of brain infarction (43% *vs* 37%) and death (22% *vs* 16%), relative to the placebo group.[45] These numbers included both symptomatic and asymptomatic haemorrhagic transformation detected by repeated CT scanning. The only clinical trial that showed superiority of thrombolysis over placebo was the National Institute of Neurological Disorders and Stroke (NINDS) sponsored study of alteplase.[46] The rate of haemorrhagic conversion was relatively low (6.4%, compared with 0.6% for placebo) because there were fewer protocol violations than in the ECASS trial,[45] and because half of the patients were treated within the first 90 minutes with a smaller alteplase dose.[46]

In the NINDS trial,[46] patients received the alteplase in a dose of 0.9 mg/kg (maximum 90mg); 10% of the dose was given in a bolus, followed by a constant intravenous infusion of the remainder over 60 minutes. The attending physicians used an algorithm to manage blood pressure with intravenous labetalol after thrombolysis began, otherwise the post-treatment elevation in blood pressure may have increased the risk of haemorrhage.[47] Patients treated with alteplase were at least 30% more likely to have minimal or no disability at 3 months on the various neurological assessment scales, compared with patients who received placebo. This trial[46] represents the first successful step towards effective and well-tolerated acute clot lysis for patients with an ischaemic stroke. Further trials are underway to evaluate other thrombolytic agents, intra-arterial delivery, and late administration of alteplase (up to 5 hours post stroke).

We have conducted our own economic evaluation of the NINDS study (Oh et al., 1996, unpublished data). We aimed to weigh the considerable added drug expenditure associated with alteplase against the significantly improved clinical outcomes and risk of serious bleeding, and need for ancillary resources, such as an intensive care unit. The higher acquisition costs of alteplase ($Can2245 per 100mg; costs to the pharmacy department, Sunnybrook Hospital, Toronto, Ontario, Canada in 1996) will be offset to some degree by decreased resource requirements for the management of disabled patients, both in the short and long term. Thus, the apparent incremental cost of the alteplase strategy might narrow to a few hundred dollars per patient and lead to a very attractive cost-effectiveness ratio per life year or QALY. Fagan et al.[48] used a Markov model to estimate costs associated with alteplase therapy in a cohort of 1000 patients. They used NINDS trial data on length of stay and concluded that direct costs of alteplase can be partially offset by a reduction in length of stay by 1.5 days in the US hospital system. Hospitals need to facilitate early discharge of patients with stroke who were treated with alteplase to achieve cost-effective allocation of resources. More precise estimates of these values will be published in the near future.

3.3.2 Impact of Thrombolytic Therapy

We have attempted to quantify the impact of thrombolytic therapy in our own institution, an academic teaching hospital. In a previous paper,[25] we detailed the costs of acute stroke care for all first admissions to our institution for 285 consecutive patients in 1991 and 1992. The average total hospital cost for a patient with a stroke totalled $Can27 500 ($Can680 per day) and was broken down into physician and medical services, nursing, occupational therapy, diagnostic testing and pharmacy costs.[25]

We illustrate this with more recent data on direct hospital costs in a patient with an acute stroke who stayed in the hospital, including the rehabilitation unit, for an extended period of 62 days (fig. 1a). We can see that in the pre-thrombolytic area, the majority of costs can be attributed to nursing care, with relatively little to pharmacy and physicians. With successful thrombolytic therapy, it might be possible to ameliorate or completely reverse severe neurological deficits. There will certainly be added costs attributable to pharmacy expenditures and early intensity of nursing care, but overall, the length of stay should shorten and this may be reflected in a reduction of the total hospitalisation costs. This is demonstrated by the breakdown of costs in a patient with minor stroke with early recovery of neurological deficit (fig. 1b). Since this patient spent only 1 day in hospital, pharmacy expenses represented 21% of the total cost (fig. 1b) compared with 4% when the length of stay was 62 days (fig. 1a).

In the thrombolytic era, the cost of alteplase would be added to the pharmacy expenses during the first day of hospital care, and the pharmacy share would increase up to 76% (fig. 1c). The projected costs for the remainder of the hospitalisation are unclear, since the NINDS trial showed only a trend towards improved neurological recovery during the first 24 hours in patients treated with alteplase.[46]

Thus, the net benefit from alteplase remains to be determined and the impact of thrombolysis on hospital resource utilisation still needs to be quantified. In our hospital, it is unlikely that any cost savings will accrue unless the average length of stay is reduced by at least 4 days, or there are savings of more than 10% of the average total direct costs,[25] in order to offset the added costs of alteplase treatment and intensive care unit expenditures. Therefore, we suggest that economic parameters, such as length of stay and intensity of resource usage, be incorporated into the analysis of future prospective trials of thrombolytic agents in order to help guide formulary and therapeutic decisions.

4. Directions for the Future

The list of risk factors for stroke is being updated, and recent results from the multinational Monitoring of Trends and Determinants in Cardiovascular

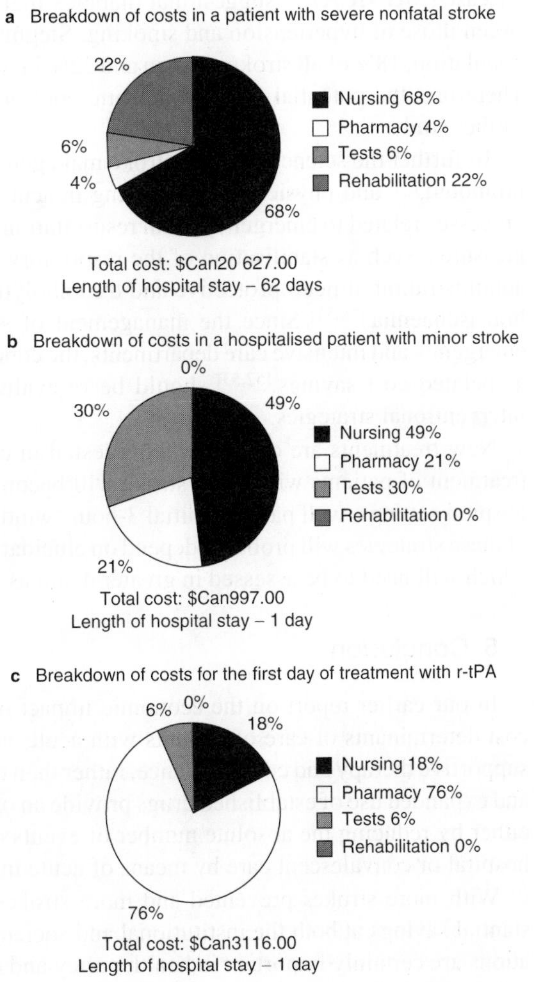

Fig. 1. Breakdown of costs for 3 hypothetical patients with stroke: (**a**) patient with severe nonfatal stroke. The patient had hemiplegia and aphasia, and required assistance in activities of daily living. The length of stay was determined by placement problems (no nursing home or relatives were immediately available) and the patient was kept at the rehabilitation unit in the hospital; (**b**) hospitalised patient with minor stroke. Minor neurological deficit was present on admission and at discharge including mild arm and leg weakness, and the patient was fully capable of self-support; and (**c**) patient with moderate neurological deficit on admission treated with alteplase (recombinant tissue plasminogen activator; r-tPA) on first day with no haemorrhagic complications. The length of stay in patients treated with alteplase depends on the rapidity of neurological improvement and costs are provided for the first day of hospital care. Additional cost of daily hospital care averages $Can680.00.[25]

Disease (MONICA)[49] suggest that diabetes mellitus is a risk factor with a magnitude between those of hypertension and smoking. Stegmayr and Asplund[49] reported that in a given population, 18% of all strokes in men and 22% in women were attributable to diabetes mellitus. Therefore, the potential of good diabetic control with regard to stroke prevention deserves further study.

To further the science of acute stroke management, the concept of a 'brain attack' has been promoted,[34] and physicians specialising in acute care are becoming more familiar with the processes related to emergency brain resuscitation; these include not only standard supportive measures, such as stabilisation of the respiratory and circulatory systems, but also the early administration of neuroprotective and thrombolytic agents within the first few hours of cerebral ischaemia.[46,51] Since the management of stroke is increasingly directed towards the emergency and intensive care departments, the concept of an acute stroke unit, and the potential associated cost savings,[52,53] should be re-evaluated, with a view to confirming effective interventional strategies.

New treatments are currently being tested in clinical trials, and it may be that multidrug treatment of patients with acute stroke will become the norm in both the prehospital and the hospital settings, well past the initial 3-hour 'window'.[54] The efficacy and cost effectiveness of these strategies will probably depend on elucidation of the pathogenic mechanisms of stroke, which will need to be assessed in greater detail as the results of these trials become available.

5. Conclusion

In our earlier report on the economic impact of stroke,[25] we emphasised that the major cost determinants of care of patients with acute stroke in Canadian hospitals were related to supportive therapy and convalescence, rather than to physician or drug costs. New medications and expanded use of established drugs provide an opportunity to have an impact on these costs, either by reducing the absolute number of events or altering the duration and nature of acute hospital or convalescent care by means of acute interventions.

With more strokes prevented and more strokes reversed, we will probably achieve substantial savings at both the institutional and societal levels. However, although cost considerations are certainly important in health policy and resource allocation, the decisions that need to be made in the case of the individual patient are certainly more difficult. Ongoing trials are warranted to find effective and safe therapies to prevent and treat ischaemic strokes in the general population.

References

1. American Heart Association. 1992 Heart and stroke facts. Dallas: American Heart Association, 1992
2. Lanska DJ, Kryscio R. Geographic distribution of hospitalization rates, case fatality, and mortality from stroke in the United States. Neurology 1995; 45: 634-40
3. Emanuel EJ, Emanuel LL. The economics of dying - the illusion of cost savings at the end of life. N Engl J Med 1994; 330: 540-4
4. Kawachi I, Malcolm LA. The cost-effectiveness of treating mild-to-moderate hypertension: a reappraisal. J Hypertension 1991; 9: 199-208
5. Rocella EJ, Lenfant C. Considerations regarding the cost and effectiveness of public and patient education programmes. J Hum Hypertens 1992; 6: 463-7
6. Gorelick PB. Stroke prevention: an opportunity for efficient utilization of health care resources during the coming decade. Stroke 1994; 25: 220-4
7. Broderick JP, Phillips SJ, Whisnant JP, et al. Incidence rates of stroke in the eighties: the end of the decline in stroke? Stroke 1989; 20: 577-82

8. Wolf PA, D'Agostino RB, O'Neal A, et al. Secular trends in stroke incidence and mortality: the Framingham study. Stroke 1992; 23: 1551-5
9. North American Symptomatic Carotid Endaretectomy Trial Collaborators. Beneficial effect of carotid endarterectomy in symptomatic patients with high grade carotid stenosis. N Engl J Med 1991; 325: 445-53
10. Executive Committee for the Asymptomatic Carotid Atherosclerosis Study. Endarterectomy for asymptomatic carotid artery stenosis. JAMA 1995; 273: 1421-8
11. Collins R, Peto R, MacMahon S, et al. Blood pressure, stroke, and coronary heart disease. Part 2. Short-term reductions in blood pressure: overview of randomized drug trials in their epidemiological context. Lancet 1990; 335: 827-38
12. Weinstein MC, Stason WB. Allocation of resources to manage hypertension. N Engl J Med 1977; 296: 732-7
13. Edelson JT, Weinstein MC, Tosteson ANA, et al. Long-term cost-effectiveness of various initial monotherapies for mild to moderate hypertension. JAMA 1990; 263: 408-13
14. Gafni A. On the costs of treating mild hypertension. J Gen Intern Med 1987; 2: 441-3
15. Millikan C, Futrell N. The strange story of aspirin and the prevention of stroke. J Stroke Cerebrovasc Dis 1995; 5: 248-54
16. Barnett HJM, Eliasziw M, Meldrum HE. Drugs and surgery in the prevention of ischemic stroke. N Engl J Med 1995; 332: 238-48
17. Solomon DH, Hart RG. Antithrombotic therapies for stroke prevention. Curr Opin Neurol 1994; 7: 48-53
18. Antiplatelet Trialists Collaboration. Collaborative overview of randomised trials of antiplatelet therapy – I: prevention of death, myocardial infarction, and stroke by prolonged antiplatelet therapy in various categories of patients. BMJ 1994; 308: 81-106
19. Hass WK, Easton JD, Adams Jr HP, et al. A randomized trial comparing ticlopidine hydrochloride with aspirin for the prevention of stroke in high-risk patients. N Engl J Med 1989; 321: 501-7
20. Oster G, Huse DM, Lacey MJ, et al. Cost-effectiveness of ticlopidine in preventing stroke in high-risk patients. Stroke 1994; 25: 1149-56
21. Van Gijn J, Algra A. Ticlopidine, trials, and torture. Stroke 1994; 25: 1097-8
22. Warlow CP. Ticlopidine, a new antithrombotic drug: but is it better than aspirin for long-term use? J Neurol Neurosurg Psychiatry 1990; 53: 185-7
23. Bladin CF, Norris JW. Relative benefits of ticlopidine and aspirin [letter]. Stroke 1994; 25: 2290
24. Roderick J, Wilkes HC, Meade TW. The gastrointestinal toxicity of aspirin: an overview of randomized controlled trials. Br J Clin Pharmacol 1993; 35: 219-26
25. Smurawska LT, Alexandrov AV, Bladin CF, et al. Cost of acute stroke care in Toronto, Canada. Stroke 1994; 25: 1628-31
26. Feinberg WM, Blackshear JL, Laupacis A, et al. Prevalence, age distribution, and gender of patients with atrial fibrillation. Arch Intern Med 1995; 155: 469-73
27. Boston Area Anticoagulation Trial for Atrial Fibrillation investigators. The effect of low-dose warfarin on the risk of stroke in patients with non-rheumatic atrial fibrillation. N Engl J Med 1990; 323: 1505-11
28. Stroke Prevention in Atrial Fibrillation investigators. Stroke prevention in atrial fibrillation study: final results. Circulation 1991; 84: 527-39
29. Gage BF, Cardinalli AB, Albers GW, et al. Cost-effectiveness of warfarin and aspirin for prophylaxis of stroke in patients with nonvalvular atrial fibrillation. JAMA 1995; 274: 1839-45
30. European Atrial Fibrillation Trial Study group. Secondary stroke prevention in non-rheumatic atrial fibrillation after transient ischaemic attack or minor stroke. Lancet 1993; 342: 1255-62
31. Petersen P, Boysen G, Godtfredsen J, et al. Placebo-controlled, randomized trial of warfarin and aspirin for prevention of thromboembolic complications in chronic atrial fibrillation: the Copenhagen AFASAK Study. Lancet 1989; II: 175-9
32. Laupacis A, Boysen G, Connolly S, et al. Risk factors for stroke and efficacy of antithrombotic therapy in atrial fibrillation. Arch Intern Med 1994; 154: 1449-57
33. Gustafsson C, Asplund K, Britton M, et al. Cost effectiveness of primary stroke prevention in atrial fibrillation: Swedish national perspective. BMJ 1992; 305: 1457-60
34. Camarata PJ, Heros RC, Latchaw RE. Brain attack: the rationale for treating stroke as a medical emergency. Neurosurgery 1994; 34: 144-58
35. Rothrock JF, Hart RG. Antithrombotic therapy in cerebrovascular disease. Arch Intern Med 1991; 115: 885-95
36. Biller J, Love BB, Gordon DE. Antithrombotic therapy for ischemic cerebrovascular disease. Semin Neurol 1991; 11: 353-67
37. The International Stroke Trial Collaborative Group. The international stroke trial. Preliminary results part II: effects of heparin [abstract]. Stroke 1997; 28: 231
38. Cerebral Embolism Study Group. Immediate anticoagulation of embolic stroke: a randomized trial. Stroke 1983; 14: 668-76
39. Duke RJ, Bloch RF, Turpie AG, et al. Intravenous heparin for prevention of stroke progression in acute partial stable stroke. Ann Intern Med 1986; 105: 825-8
40. Kay R, Wong KS, Yu YL, et al. Low-molecular-weight heparin for the treatment of acute ischemic stroke. N Engl J Med 1995; 333: 1588-93
41. Kay R, Woo J, Kreel L, et al. Stroke subtypes among Chinese living in Hong Kong: the Shatei stroke registry. Neurology 1992; 42: 985-7
42. Multicenter Acute Stroke Trial – Europe Study Group. Thrombolytic therapy with streptokinase in acute ischemic stroke. N Engl J Med 1996; 335: 145-50
43. Donnan G, Davis SM, Chambers BR, et al. Trials of streptokinase in severe acute ischaemic stroke [letter]. Lancet 1995; 345: 578-9

44. Multicentre Acute Stroke Trial – Italy (MAST-I) Group. Randomized controlled trial of streptokinase, aspirin, and combination of both in treatment of acute ischaemic stroke. Lancet 1995; 346: 1509-14
45. Hacke W, Kaste M, Fieschi C, et al. Intravenous thrombolysis with recombinant tissue plasminogen activator for acute hemispheric stroke: the European Cooperative Acute Stroke Study (ECASS). JAMA 1995; 274: 1017-25
46. National Institute of Neurological Disorders and Stroke rt-PA Stroke Study Group. Tissue plasminogen activator for acute ischemic stroke. N Engl J Med 1995; 333: 1581-7
47. Levy DE, Brott TG, Haley Jr EC, et al. Factors related to hematoma formation in patients receiving tissue-type plasminogen activator for acute ischemic stroke. Stroke 1994; 25: 291-7
48. Fagan S, Morgenstern LB, Petitta A, et al. rt-PA Reduces length of stay and improves disposition following stroke [abstract]. Stroke 1997; 28: 272
49. Stegmayr B, Asplund K. Diabetes as a risk factor for stroke: a population perspective. Diabetologia 1995; 38: 1061-8
51. Working Group on Emergency Brain Resuscitation. Emergency Brain Resuscitation. Ann Intern Med 1995; 122: 622-7
52. Langehorn P, Williams BO, Gilchrist W, et al. Do stroke units save lives? Lancet 1993; 342: 395-8
53. Jorgensen HS, Nakayama H, Raaschou HO, et al. The effect of a stroke unit: reductions in mortality, discharge rate to nursing home, length of stay, and cost. A community-based study. Stroke 1995; 26: 1178-82
54. Baron JC, von Kummer R, del Zoppo GL. Treatment of acute ischemic stroke: challenging the concept of a rigid and universal time window. Stroke 1995; 26: 2219-21

Correspondence: Dr *Andrei V. Alexandrov*, Stroke Program, University of Texas at Houston, 6431 Fannin St MSB 7.044, Houston, TX 77030, USA.